How to do a Systematic Literature Review in Nursing

A step-by-step guide

Second edition

How to do a Systematic Literature Review in Nursing

A step-by-step guide

Second edition

Josette Bettany–Saltikov and Robert McSherry

Open University Press

Open University Press
McGraw-Hill Education
8th Floor
338 Euston Road
London
England
NW1 3BT

email: enquiries@openup.co.uk
world wide web: www.openup.co.uk

and Two Penn Plaza, New York, NY 10121-2289, USA

First published 2012
Second edition published 2016

A catalogue record of this book is available from the British Library

ISBN-13: 978-0-33-526380-6
ISBN-10: 0-33-526380-1
eISBN: 978-0-33-526381-3

Library of Congress Cataloging-in-Publication Data
CIP data applied for

Typeset by SPi-Global

Printed by Bell and Bain Ltd, Glasgow

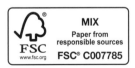

MIX
Paper from
responsible sources
FSC® C007785

Praise page

"This is a valuable text that will prove useful for nurses who are planning to write a systematic review of the literature, whether as part of an academic assignment or for publication.
The book is clearly written, easy to follow and comprehensive, taking readers through all of the key steps in a literature review. It offers a range of case studies and examples that will help to contextualise and clarify the steps of a review.

The authors also signpost readers to a variety of resources and provide practical tips, summaries and templates to work through as part of the review process. This will be an important text for undergraduate and post-graduate nurses and I thoroughly recommend it."
> *Professor Fiona Irvine, Head of Nursing, University of Birmingham, UK*

"This book is a very comprehensive, well written and illustrated key text on systematic reviews for anyone involved in research within nursing. Its strengths are its well laid-out format, mixing figures and tables with real examples throughout. It is a key resource for both the novice and more advanced researcher and will be a major support to students from basic degree right up to PhD level."
> *Dr. Pauline Joyce, Academic Co-ordinator, RCSI School of Medicine, Ireland*

"This timely second edition of this book will form a core text for many nursing and healthcare students and their lecturers. The book provides a highly practical, thorough and logical overview to enable even novices to undertake a systematic literature review. Unlike some other methodological texts, the book is written in an easily accessible style, yet provides the necessary theoretical underpinning presented in a non-threatening way. The reader is directed to useful resources and the Q&A sections that follow the chapter summaries are helpful for students to self-assess their learning. The key points keep the reader on track, and helpful practical tips are woven into the text throughout. It's a great book!"
> *Dr. Debbie Roberts, Professor in Nurse Education and*
> *Clinical Learning, and Head of the Research Centre for*
> *the School of Social and Life Sciences, Glyndwr University, UK*

Dedication

We would like to dedicate this second edition to our parents (Josette – Francis and Marcelle Damato; Robert – Dorothy and Wilfred McSherry) who unfortunately are not alive today but who are in our thoughts every day.

We would like to dedicate this book to all our past and present undergraduate and postgraduate students for all their words of encouragement and support in inspiring and motivating us both to produce this second edition.

Finally we dedicate this book to all our family and friends for your continued love, support and belief in what we do every day.

Contents

List of boxes

List of figures

List of tables

Foreword

Sometimes in my imagination I like to think about what it must have been like to nurse in times past. In these dreams I go to somewhere like pre-European Australia. A "nurse", perhaps a wise woman, would have been an observant person. She would have noted during her life, the cycle of the seasons, the cycle of birth and death and the cycles of illnesses. Some ailments such as fevers, diarrhoea or infected wounds may have become familiar, their natural course known. This nurse may also have known of remedies and practices, passed down from generations of other wise, observant people. She would have used this knowledge to treat these aliments and care for the sick; the bark of a particular tree to soothe a fever, a particular technique to reduce a fractured limb, practices to comfort a sick child, or a poultice of a plant to ward off wound infection. Some of these practices are now being rediscovered today and subjected to research.

Living a nomadic lifestyle in small groups over a vast continent it may have taken centuries for such knowledge to accumulate and even longer for this evidence to spread. Even then the natural resources relied upon for some remedies would differ markedly over a continent whose environments range from snow covered mountains, dense tropical rainforest to stony deserts. Not all of the practices and remedies always worked. Nevertheless, I imagine our nursing ancestor to be a keen observer of cause and effect, and who, given the resources and knowledge available to her, used the best available evidence to care for the sick.

Today's nurses are also keen observers and keen to do the best they can for the patients for whom they care. Given the advent of hospitals we are better able to understand the natural history of various diseases as we are able to observe and compare thousands of similar cases. We are also able to devise rigorous qualitative and quantitative research to answer important questions of effectiveness, appropriateness and meaningfulness in relation to our nursing care. However, this evidence remains scattered and isolated like the knowledge accumulated by our nursing ancestors unless we can find ways of synthesising these research findings and rendering them useful for practice. The crop of nursing research continues to grow, and we now need to harvest the evidence and kneed it into a useful dough that can form the basis of our care.

To stretch the food metaphor a little further, it is therefore fitting that this book details in "bite size" chunks the step by step processes of how to systematically review the body of nursing knowledge. The book is commendably readable and practical, the authors have avoided impenetrable language and the book is replete with examples from practice. Most importantly, Josette Bettany-Saltikov and Rob McSherry have carried on a proud tradition of nursing; finding ways to provide the best care possible to our communities and thereby positively impact on global health.

Professor Kenneth Walsh, RN PhD, Fellow of the Joanna Briggs Institute.
Professor of Translational Research in Nursing and Midwifery,
School of Health Sciences, University of Tasmania, and the Tasmanian Health Service.
Hobart, Australia.

Acknowledgements

We would like to personally thank our students for kindly giving their permission to use extracts from their dissertations to allow us to illustrate by example through the case studies within the book. We would also like to thank all of our undergraduate and postgraduate students for their words of encouragement for writing this second edition. We have learned as much from you as we hope you have from us. We would also like to thank Caldwell et al. (2011) for kindly allowing and permitting us to use their framework. Finally, we would like to thank our colleagues and the publishing team for their support and encouragement through the second journey of creating this book.

Introduction

We are very pleased to provide this second edition of *How to Do A Systematic Literature Review in Nursing: A Step-by-Step Guide.* We hope you find the second edition as equally useful and practical as the first. The revisions and enhancements to this edition are based on individual feedback and from published reviews. We also had the first edition sent for independent peer review to five leads for research within academic institutions across the United Kingdom. We would like to personally thank these reviewers and all individuals who have so kindly taken the time to provide feedback in helping us to reshape the second edition.

Since the first publication of the book we have noticed that the popularity of undertaking a systematic review within undergraduate and postgraduate nursing and allied health professions educational programmes is increasing. They are forming part of undergraduate dissertations, fulfilling assessment criteria for research and evidence-based nursing modules, forming part of the final dissertation modules to fulfil the requirements of Masters and Doctoral Degrees. Perhaps the reasons for this are in light of issues associated with achieving ethical approval and/or undertaking live research in a relatively short fixed period of time – or simply a desire to answer a burning clinical question from practice.

You will notice that we have updated the book to provide an even more step-by-step guide by increasing the chapters from 9 to 12. We have done this to help simplify some of the existing information into more 'bite-sized chunks'. We have included some additional case studies, practical tips and question and answers and retained the 'key points' sections – all aiming to enhance the progression and quality of your systematic review. We have also included templates to enable you to undertake each part of the systematic literature review process with confidence.

The aim of the book is to continue to provide a simple and practical step-by-step approach to conducting a systematic literature review. We have tried as much as possible to present all the content in this book in a simple and clear format in order to make it suitable for your own abilities and level of learning. This book is intended for all nurses in practice, nursing students and nurse lecturers teaching at universities as well as other healthcare professionals in a diverse range of settings.

A conversational style has purposely been retained because several reviews indicated that this was a key strength of the first edition and was successful in engaging the reader as much as possible. We would like to encourage and not discourage you in seeing the value of undertaking a systemic review and how this may lead to improvements in patient safety, quality and compassionate care and services in the future. We know from our own experience, our students' experience and from undertaking research surrounding evidence-based nursing that some nurses and student nurses are put off research if the content that is presented is very academic and full of jargon. We are of the opinion that a systematic literature review (or systematic review) is not only for doctors or high-level Cochrane review researchers. We have found over the past several years that anyone with basic undergraduate research skills is capable of undertaking this type of review. We can say this confidently because we have taught this method of reviewing to nurses and nursing students over many years.

When we have taught about systematic literature reviews and the term systematic review is mentioned, many students started panicking and saying 'I don't know how to do this!' But our combined experience of having taught over 800 students on a number of dissertation modules has proved that once the individual steps are shown to learners in a straight-forward manner, all levels of students including undergraduate nurses, Masters and Doctoral students, returning nurses, nurse specialists and practitioners are indeed able and capable of undertaking a systematic review to completion and to a high standard. Some students have even published their systematic literature review.

This second edition continues to offer a practical guide that you can use to support you step-by-step from start to completion of your own systematic literature review. We hope you enjoy this second edition of the book and that you are successful with undertaking your systematic review. The following contains an overview of the contents of the book:

Chapter 1: What is a systematic review?

This chapter introduces the term 'systematic review'. The different types of systematic reviews and common databases for finding these reviews are discussed. Their role within evidence-based nursing practice, as well as the differences between literature (narrative) reviews and systematic ones are then debated and the medical hierarchy of evidence briefly described.

Chapter 2: Asking an answerable and focused review question

In this chapter the key points to remember when selecting a review topic are described and different ways of narrowing the review topic to a specific question presented. This is followed by a discussion of the meaning and functions of an answerable and focused review question. The main types of focused research questions are then discussed and some examples from nursing practice are provided. This is followed by a presentation on the different types of research questions and the importance of selecting the appropriate research design for the type of research question you have selected. A number of templates are also provided to help you formulate your own answerable and focused review question.

Chapter 3: Creating the protocol for your systematic review

This chapter highlights the importance of writing a protocol for your review, the steps to take and sections to be included within your protocol. The importance of managing and planning your time is highlighted.

Chapter 4: Writing the background to your review

This chapter details the background information required to prepare your protocol providing an operational definition of the clinical problem. The importance of the review question and grabbing the attention of the reader is highlighted. Issues associated with clarifying the gap in systematic reviews in the clinical area are discussed and how to apply different tools and methods to help you start writing up your background section.

Chapter 5: Specifying your objectives and inclusion and exclusion criteria

This chapter discusses the meanings and differences between a problem statement, an aim, an objective as well as a review question. Methods for specifying the inclusion and exclusion criteria are discussed and examples provided for different quantitative and qualitative review questions. Templates are also provided to help readers write out their own problem statement, aims and objectives as well as their inclusion and exclusion criteria.

Chapter 6: Conducting a comprehensive and systematic literature search

This chapter discusses the importance, the rational as well as the aims of undertaking a comprehensive and systematic search. The key factors to be considered when undertaking a comprehensive search are described as well as the steps involved in converting your review question into a comprehensive search strategy.

Chapter 7: Working with your primary papers: Stage 1 – Selecting the studies to include in your systematic review

This chapter discusses working with your primary papers (stage 1) associated with selecting the appropriate papers to answer your review question and the methods of the review. The templates to select the papers for your own systematic literature review are detailed.

Chapter 8: Working with your primary papers: Stage 2 – Appraising the methodological quality of your included research studies

The chapter details working with your primary papers (stage 2) appraising the methodological quality of your included research studies. The methods of the review, appraising the methodological quality of the research papers that you have selected and a worked example of using the Caldwell et al. framework to critique a nursing paper are provided.

Chapter 9: Working with your primary papers: Stage 3 – Extracting the data from your included papers

The chapter details working with your primary papers (stage 3) associated with extracting data from your included papers. The methods of review and how to extract the appropriate data from your included research papers are discussed.

Chapter 10: Synthesizing, summarizing and presenting your findings

This chapter discusses issues to consider when synthesizing and summarizing your results. The tools to use when summarizing and synthesizing your results are offered and ways of how and where to get started on presenting your results detailed. The ways of presenting the results of your search, the results of the studies selected based on the title and abstract, the results of the studies selected based on reading the full paper, a summary of all your included studies, a summary of all the critiques of your included papers using the appropriate frameworks and summary of the data extracted (including a synthesis of the overall results) are offered. Summarizing, synthesizing and presenting your interventions and comparative interventions, outcomes and quantitative and qualitative outcome measures are discussed.

Chapter 11: Writing up your discussion and completing your review

This chapter discusses ways of structuring the 'discussion section' of your systematic literature review. Extracts from case studies as well as a completed systematic review are presented and debated. Suggestions for writing up your review report are also described, as are tips for improving academic writing skills.

Chapter 12: Checking your systematic review is complete and some practical ways to share and disseminate your findings

This chapter provides a systematic review checklist with explanations, the preferred reporting items for systematic reviews and meta-analysis (PRISMA) statements and some practical ways to help support you in sharing and disseminating your systematic literature review.

1

What is a systematic review?

Overview

- What is a systematic review?
- What is the purpose of systematic reviews within nursing practice?
- What is the role of systematic reviews within evidence-based nursing practice?
- What is the difference between a literature (narrative) review and a systematic review?
- What is the difference between a systematic review and a meta-analysis?
- What are the different types of reviews that can be found in the literature?
- Where can I find systematic reviews?
- What are the drawbacks and limitations of systematic reviews?

What is a systematic review?

A systematic review is a summary of the research literature that is focused on a single question. It is conducted in a manner that tries to identify, select, appraise and synthesize all high-quality research evidence relevant to that question. High-quality research includes those studies with an explicit and rigorous design that allow the findings to be interrogated against clear contexts and research intentions. When conducting systematic reviews, we need to accept that there is a hierarchy of evidence and that what can confidently be stated *empirically* about the world is derived from studies where the design is both explicit and rigorous. Distinctions are therefore made between 'evidence' and 'experience'. The first has been rigorously obtained and scrutinized; the latter has simply been noted, organized and reported. An understanding of systematic reviews and how to implement them in practice is now becoming mandatory for all nurses and other healthcare professionals as part of standards for professional practice (Health and Care Professionals Council 2012, Centre for Evidence-Based Medicine 2015, Nursing and Midwifery Council 2015).

The National Institute for Health Research (NIHR) in the United Kingdom (UK) is a global leader in producing and promoting systematic reviews. They produce high-quality research evidence that supports decision-making in all aspects of health and social care. The NIHR (2010: 2) states that 'Systematic reviews identify, evaluate, combine and summarise the findings of all relevant individual studies and provide decision-makers with the best possible information about the effects of tests, treatments and other interventions used in health and social care'.

What is the purpose of systematic reviews within nursing practice?

The Centre for Reviews and Dissemination (University of York) states:

> Healthcare decisions for individual patients and for public policy should be informed by the best available research evidence. Practitioners and decision-makers are encouraged to make use of the latest research and information about best practice, and to ensure that decisions are demonstrably rooted in this knowledge.
>
> (Centre for Reviews and Dissemination 2008: v)

Following this advice can sometimes be difficult for nurse practitioners and researchers because of the large amount of information published in a multitude of journals worldwide. Individual research studies may be *biased* or methodologically unsound and can reach conflicting conclusions. Examples of conflicting research results are frequently found in the media, which may announce that based on the research results of the latest study, the contraceptive pill is 'safe', and then a week later proclaim the exact opposite based on the results of another research study. In such situations it is not always clear which results are the most reliable, or which should be used as the basis of policy and practice decisions (Petticrew and Roberts 2006).

A systematic review should also be based on a peer-review protocol (or plan) so that it can be easily replicated if necessary. The review itself will include a 'background' or introduction, in which the authors explain the scientific background or context to their study. It also includes the rationale for the systematic review indicating why it is necessary. The specific objectives and a summary of how the reviewer defined the criteria by which to choose the research papers are stated. Once a thorough assessment of the quality of each included research paper or report is carried out, all the individual studies are synthesized in an unbiased way. The findings are then interpreted and presented in an objective and independent summary (Hemmingway and Brereton 2009).

Systematic reviews are used by a wide diversity of professional and non-professional groups, including not only doctors, nurses and other healthcare professionals but also service users, policy-makers, researchers, lecturers and students who want to keep up with the sometimes overwhelming amount of evidence in their field. It is important that nurses have the research skills to both understand and undertake systematic reviews, because they may want to know the answer to a clinical or research question or they may be conducting a systematic review in a dissertation required to complete a degree or as a continuing professional development requirement. Conducting a systematic review can initially appear to be an epic task, but once the steps of the process are learnt, and provided enough time is set aside, the task is relatively straightforward.

How difficult is it to undertake a systematic review?

Having taught large numbers of students about how to conduct this type of review on dissertation modules, we are confident that both undergraduate and postgraduate students can competently undertake and complete this type of review to a satisfactory level.

If this is the first time you are undertaking this type of review, ensure that you carry it out in small steps and allow sufficient time to work on all the stages of the systematic review. It is important to understand that systematic reviews can be undertaken only on primary research papers. It is not possible to conduct a systematic review using other types of studies such as narrative reviews or opinion papers.

The three main types of systematic reviews are quantitative, qualitative and mixed method reviews. Quantitative systematic reviews generally include only quantitative primary research studies whereas qualitative systematic reviews include only qualitative primary research studies. Mixed method reviews are based on both qualitative and quantitative studies; they are becoming more common nowadays, although they may be a bit more difficult to conduct. For the purposes of simplicity, this book will consider only the quantitative and qualitative types of reviews.

There are several sources available for finding systematic reviews. These include the Joanna Briggs Institute (JBI) (http://joannabriggs.org/), Centre for Reviews and Dissemination (The University of York, https://www.york.ac.uk/crd/) and the Cochrane Library (http://www.cochranelibrary.com), which is one of the best known sources for finding quantitative systematic reviews. The Cochrane Library concentrates mainly on synthesizing the findings of randomized controlled trials (RCTs). There is also a qualitative Cochrane Review database and the Campbell Collaboration database, where numerous qualitative systematic reviews can be found. Many systematic reviews are also published in key professional nursing journals. Some examples include the following.

- **Primary Care** – 'The management of urinary incontinence and promotion of continence using conservative behavioural approaches in older people in care homes' (Roe et al. 2015).
- **Adult Nursing** – 'Non-cancer palliative care in the community needs greater interprofessional collaboration to maintain coordinated care and manage uncertainty' (de Brito and Gommes 2015).
- **Professional Development** – 'Measuring the Effectiveness of Mentoring as a Knowledge Translation Intervention for Implementing Empirical Evidence: A Systematic Review' (Abdullah et al. 2014).

Practical Tip

Systematic reviews are a sound way of keeping up to date with the latest evidence surrounding a specific area and aspect of nursing. Systematic reviews are regularly updated and are current sources of evidence.

What is the role of systematic reviews within evidence-based nursing practice?

The popularity of evidence-based practice has increased significantly since the mid-1990s, when Sackett et al. (1997) first coined the term. For a nurse to practise evidence-based nursing DiCenso et al. comment:

A nurse has to decide whether the evidence is relevant for the particular patient. The incorporation of clinical expertise should be balanced with the risks and benefits of alternative treatments for each patient and should take into account the patient's unique clinical circumstances including comorbid conditions and preferences.

(DiCenso et al. 1998: 38)

It is important to think about what is meant by the *best* research evidence. Within evidence-based practice there is a hierarchy of research evidence relating to studies with different types of research designs. This hierarchy has systematic reviews at the top and qualitative studies and opinion papers towards the bottom (Table 1.1). The hierarchy of evidence is a medically based model that is considered by some professional groups to be biased towards quantitative research and intervention studies. Although qualitative studies are found at the bottom, it is important to consider that they answer very different types of questions relating to patient experiences. A number of authors and researchers have objected to the classification in Table 1.1, stating that this model does not accurately represent the high-quality, qualitative research studies that inform policy and practice and that perhaps better represent patient experiences and preferences.

Table 1.1 Levels of evidence for different types of research questions

Level 1a	A well-conducted systematic review of randomized controlled trials (RCTs)
Level 1b	One good quality RCT
Level 1c	All or none studies
Level 2a	Systematic review of cohort studies
Level 2b	One cohort study
Level 2c	Outcomes research, i.e. the effect of an intervention or treatment
Level 3a	Systematic review of case-control studies
Level 3b	Case series
Level 4	One case study
Level 5	Qualitative studies and expert opinion

Note: The research questions can include nursing interventions, therapy, prevention, aetiology (causes) or harm.

The traditional scientific approach to finding the best research evidence is to carry out or read a literature review (conducted by an expert or well-known figure in the field). However, these traditional (or narrative) reviews, even those written by experts, can be made to tell any story one wants them to and failure by literature reviewers to apply scientific principles to the process of reviewing, just as one would to primary research, can lead to biased conclusions, harm to patients and wasted resources (Petticrew and Roberts 2006: 5).

Craig and Smyth (2007: 185) state: 'Because systematic reviews include a comprehensive search strategy, appraisal and synthesis of research evidence, they can be used as shortcuts in the evidence-based process'. Systematic reviews provide practitioners with a way of gaining access to predigested evidence. According to Petticrew and Roberts (2006: 9), systematic reviews 'adhere closely to a set of scientific methods that explicitly aim to limit systematic error (bias), mainly attempting to identify, appraise and synthesize all relevant studies (of whatever design) in order *to answer a particular question (or set of questions)*' (our emphasis). Systematic reviews substantially reduce the time and expertise it would take to locate, appraise and synthesize individual studies.

What is the difference between a literature (narrative) review and a systematic review?

Traditional literature (narrative) reviews can, as already mentioned, tell any story that the reviewer wants them to (Glasziou et al. 2001). For example, if the reviewer is a strong believer in the effectiveness of aspirin for treating headaches but does not believe that any other medication is effective, this reviewer could (hypothetically) select all the papers showing the effectiveness of aspirin and leave out all the ones showing the effectiveness of, say, ibuprofen.

While both traditional (narrative) and systematic reviews provide summaries of the available literature on a topic, they fulfil very different needs. Although narrative reviews (also called critical reviews) provide valuable summaries by experts on a wide topic area, they usually present an *overview*. These types of reviews do not usually follow a scientific review methodology and the papers included can be haphazard and biased. Nevertheless, they can be an important source of ideas, arguments, context and information. Narrative reviews are valuable because they are written by experts in the field and provide a general summary of the topic area, but they may not always include all the literature on the topic and sometimes they may be biased in terms of which articles are selected and discussed (Petticrew and Roberts 2006).

Narrative reviewers can be influenced by their preferred theories, needs and beliefs. It is important to remember that narrative reviews are usually driven by a general interest in a topic and *not* directed by a stated question. Narrative reviews do not state the criteria that determine the search undertaken and can be disorganized. A notorious example is the review conducted by the eminent doctor, Linus Pauling (1974), who was a Nobel prize laureate. In 1974, having conducted a non-systematic traditional review, he concluded that people should be getting 100 times the amount of vitamin C that the food and nutrition board recommended at the time; he suggested that such doses could *prevent* a cold. Some 30 years later Douglas et al. (2004) conducted a thorough systematic review of papers from the same period as Pauling's review; they concluded that high doses of vitamin C *did not prevent* colds (although this could reduce the duration by one or two days). Douglas et al. (2004) found that Pauling had failed to include 15 relevant studies in his review. It is therefore important to remember that 'a haphazard review, even one carried out by an expert, can be misleading' (Petticrew and Roberts 2006: 6).

A systematic review in contrast uses *a rigorous research methodology* to try to limit bias in all aspects of the review. In this sense it is close to a primary research study, where the participants are not people but rather the papers included in the review. Khan et al. (2003: 1) suggest that 'a systematic review is a research article that identifies relevant studies, appraises their quality and summarizes their results using a scientific methodology'. Table 1.2 summarizes the differences and similarities between the two types of reviews.

Table 1.2 Similarities and differences between a narrative review and a systematic review

	Systematic reviews	*Narrative reviews*
Question	Focused on a single question	Not necessarily focused on a single question but may describe an overview of a topic
Protocol	A peer-review protocol (or plan) is included	No protocol
Background/literature review	Both provide summaries of the available literature on a topic	
Objectives	Has clear objectives stated	Objectives may or may not be identified
Inclusion/exclusion criteria	Criteria stated before the review is conducted	Criteria not usually specified
Search strategy	Comprehensive search conducted in a systematic way	Search strategy not explicitly stated
Process of selecting papers	Selection process usually clear and explicit	Selection process not described
Process of evaluating papers	Comprehensive evaluation of study quality	Evaluation of study quality may or may not be included
Process of extracting relevant information	Process is usually clear and specific	Process of extracting relevant information is not explicit and clear
Results/data synthesis	Clear summaries of studies based on high-quality evidence	Summary based on studies where the quality of included papers may not be specified, and can be influenced by reviewers' pet theories, needs and beliefs
Discussion	Written by an expert or group of experts with a detailed and well-grounded knowledge of the issues	

What is the difference between a systematic review and a meta-analysis?

As described above, a systematic review is a thorough, comprehensive and explicit way of evaluating the nursing literature. It is a summary of the research literature that is focused on a single question. It is conducted in a manner that tries to identify, select, appraise and synthesize all high-quality research evidence relevant to that question. A systematic review may or may not include a meta-analysis.

A 'meta-analysis' is a statistical approach to combine the data derived from a systematic review. Therefore, every meta-analysis should be based on an underlying systematic review, but not every systematic review leads to a meta-analysis.

What are the different types of reviews that can be found in the literature?

See Table 1.3 for the different types of reviews that can be found in the literature

Table 1.3 Different types of reviews found in the literature

Label	Description
Rapid review	A brief version of a systematic review to search and critically appraise existing research
Scoping review	This is a brief review, the aim of which is to identify the potential size and scope of the available research literature
Critical review	This term is usually used interchangeably with the term narrative review
Mixed studies review or mixed methods review	These types of reviews combine both quantitative and qualitative reviewing, to produce the systematic review
Qualitative systematic review/qualitative evidence synthesis	This type of review synthesizes the findings from qualitative studies. It looks for 'themes' or 'lie across' individual qualitative studies
Overview	Summary of the (medical) literature that attempts to survey the literature and describe its characteristics
Umbrella review	Synthesis and summary of evidence from a group of reviews
Aggregative review	Reviews are synthesized by adding up (aggregating/counting) data to answer review questions
Configurative review	Reviews are associated with organizing and arranging data. These are usually but not always associated with qualitative data; in some instances, quantitative data can be organized and configured too

Where can I find systematic reviews?

Systematic reviews can be found in a number of different nursing journals and specialist websites. Box 1.1 provides some useful websites to start searching for systematic reviews.

Box 1.1   Websites for finding systematic reviews

- Evidence-Based Nursing (EBN):
  http://ebn.bmj.com
- TRIP database:
  www.tripdatabase.com
- Evidence in Health and Social Care:
  https://www.evidence.nhs.uk/
- Centre for Reviews and Dissemination (CRD):
  www.york.ac.uk/crd/
- Campbell Collaboration:
  www.campbellcollaboration.org
- Cochrane Library:
  www.thecochranelibrary.com
- Cochrane Qualitative & Implementation Methods Group:
  http://qim.cochrane.org/
- UK Cochrane Centre:
  www.uk.cochrane.org
- Cochrane Collaboration:
  http://www.cochrane.org/
- School of Health and Related Research (ScHARR):
  https://www.sheffield.ac.uk/scharr
- Systematic Reviews Journal:
  http://www.systematicreviewsjournal.com/
- The Evidence for Policy and Practice Information and Co-ordinating Centre (EPPI Centre):
  http://eppi.ioe.ac.uk/cms/Default.aspx?tabid=63

In the UK, the UK Cochrane Centre supports the preparation of systematic reviews of the effects of healthcare interventions produced by 22 NIHR-funded Cochrane Review Groups. As it states on their website 'the reviews are updated regularly, ensuring that treatment decisions can be based on the most up-to-date and reliable evidence' (Cochrane Collaboration 2014: para 2). Other databases where systematic reviews as well as ongoing reviews can be registered and found include the following.

- *PROSPERO* (http://www.crd.york.ac.uk/PROSPERO/). This is an open access international prospective register of systematic reviews in health and social care.
- The Health Technology Assessment (*HTA database*) collates information on completed and ongoing health technology assessments from over 70 international

agencies. The reviews independently assess the existing evidence base on the benefits, harms and costs of particular healthcare treatments and tests for those who plan, provide or receive care in the National Health Service (NHS).

- The Centre for Reviews and Dissemination also maintains access to Database of Abstracts of Reviews of Effects (*DARE*) and the NHS Economic Evaluation Database (*NHS EED*). These databases contain quality assessed systematic reviews and economic evaluations of health and social care interventions published between 1994 and 2014. From April 2015, the Centre changed its name and it is now called the *NIHR Dissemination Centre* where available summaries of new research are available.

What are the drawbacks and limitations of systematic reviews?

Although systematic reviews can be found at the top of the hierarchy of evidence, this does not mean that we should always believe the results presented within them. Like any other piece of research, a systematic review can be conducted badly, so it is important to have the skills to be able to appraise them (see Chapters 6–12). Systematic reviews may also be biased in the way they select their papers, for instance if they have not included all the primary research papers available. Sometimes systematic reviews include only English language papers and ignore all non-English language papers, which may have found different results.

Other types of biases can occur in the way that reviewers search for their research papers. If the reviewers did not conduct a comprehensive search drawing on the most relevant databases, searching for grey literature and hand searching, it is possible that a number of key papers may have been left out. Furthermore, systematic reviews may not have properly combined the results of different studies appropriately and so ended up presenting inaccurate results.

It is crucial to appraise a systematic review properly before using the results. To do this you need to ask a series of questions to evaluate if the review in question conducted all the steps in the process correctly and with minimal bias.

Key points

- A systematic review is a research article that identifies a specific review question, identifies all relevant studies, appraises their quality and summarizes their results using a scientific methodology.
- It is possible to conduct systematic reviews of many different types of primary research studies.
- Sources for finding systematic reviews include the Cochrane Library, Campbell Collaboration, the Cochrane Qualitative Research Group and key nursing journals, among others.
- Systematic reviews are based on research evidence and the synthesis of research studies and can also be used to inform important policies that affect both the quality as well as the safety and value of healthcare.
- Because systematic reviews include a comprehensive search strategy, appraisal and synthesis of research evidence, they can be used as shortcuts in the evidence-based process.

- Both traditional (narrative) and systematic reviews provide summaries of the available literature on a topic but fulfil very different needs.

- Narrative reviews provide valuable summaries by experts on a wide topic area and they usually present an *overview*.

- Narrative reviews do not follow a scientific review methodology and the papers included within them can be haphazard and biased, usually through the opinion of the study authors.

Summary

This chapter introduced the term 'systematic review' and discussed the purpose of these types of reviews within nursing research and practice. The chapter discussed different types of systematic reviews and common databases for finding them. Their role within evidence-based nursing practice and the differences between literature (narrative) reviews and systematic reviews were debated and the medical hierarchy of evidence briefly discussed. The chapter concluded by discussing the drawbacks and limitations of systematic reviews.

Question and Answer (Q&A)

(Q) Why do nurses working in the frontline need to understand about systematic reviews?

(A) Systematic reviews are an excellent way of finding answers to problems. Systematic reviews are a good way of keeping up to date with the latest evidence and in practising using an evidence base.

2

Asking an answerable and focused review question

Overview

- Selecting a topic area for your systematic review
- Narrowing the topic area to a specific answerable review question
- Using background or foreground questions: what is the difference?
- Factors to consider when asking answerable and focused review questions
- Developing your review question further
- Relating your question to the research design: what types of study designs should you look for to answer your research question?
- Relating a specific research question to an appropriate research design

Selecting a topic area for your systematic review

Selecting a topic area for your systematic review is the first step towards undertaking the review. The specific topic you select may arise from a number of different triggers. If you are a nursing student, your interest in a topic may result from a lecture or module on a nursing condition that was covered in your undergraduate classes or a nursing problem that you or a relative have experienced. The topic area may also arise from a contemporary issue highlighted in the media, such as reports on the latest research studies conducted on falls or pressure sore prevention, or nursing interventions associated with keeping patients safe, for example ensuring they are well-nourished as opposed to malnourished, or avoiding medication errors. If you are a practising nurse, it is likely that the topic area you choose is related to your professional practice, clinical working environment or a Nursing and Midwifery Council (NMC) issue or national initiative. Whatever your role and responsibility, it is important that when selecting a research topic you bear in mind a number of key points (Box 2.1).

Box 2.1   Key points to remember when choosing a research topic

When choosing a research topic, you will need to identify:

- an area you are interested in related to your practice
- a question that you would like to know the answer to
- why the question is interesting and worth investigating
- issues relating to the question
- what you will gain by investigating the question
- what your profession and other professions will gain
- the rationale for asking the question
- the use of having the answer, i.e. ask 'So what?'
- the lack of knowledge in the area
- an awareness of how the research question may improve safety, quality and practice.

Practical Tip

To help identify an appropriate research question try focusing on an aspect of nursing practice that may arise from a thank you letter, incident, event and/or aspects of the clinical environment or professional practice that are highly topical and recurring situations. You may also consider those issues that are regularly discussed and debated in multidisciplinary team and/or clinical meetings.

Narrowing the topic area to a specific answerable review question

Once you have selected your research topic or area, the next step is to narrow this down to a review question. This process is similar to a funnel or an inverted triangle (see Figure 2.1), where the wide base of the funnel represents the research topic and the narrow peak represents the specific research question. To illustrate this, a student nurse who is interested in the area of spinal deformities might select spinal deformities as the topic area, and one specific question arising from this specific topic could be 'the effectiveness of braces for treating patients with scoliosis'. Here the nurse has narrowed the topic area by specifying the particular treatment and also specifying the type of spinal deformity. Another nurse working in the accident and emergency (A&E) department may be very interested in the area of witnessed resuscitation (where family members are present during resuscitation attempts), as she has participated in a number of these procedures during her routine practice. 'Witnessed resuscitation' would then be the general topic area and a possible research (or review) question arising from this area could be 'What are the views of nurses regarding witnessed resuscitation in the A&E department?' Here the nurse has narrowed the topic area to a research question by specifying that she will be looking at nurses' views on this topic and will be restricting the study to the A&E department.

You may be asking how you actually derive the question from the topic. The way to do this is to ask a series of questions to narrow the topic down. To illustrate how

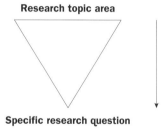

Figure 2.1 Deriving the research question from the topic area.

this is done, we will use a hypothetical case study of a spinal nurse, Cheryl. Once you have read the case study you can try to narrow down your own topic area to a review question using the template provided in Box 2.2.

Case study: spinal nurse Cheryl

Cheryl is a spinal nurse working in a new spinal unit. As part of her role in the spinal deformity department she takes care of many teenagers who suddenly develop a spinal deformity when they reach their teens, a condition known as adolescent idiopathic scoliosis (AIS). Before developing this deformity, when they were children, their spine was normal. The cause for this problem is not yet known so the treatment is concentrated on the symptoms. One of the treatments that Cheryl is involved in is bracing of the spinal curvatures to try to reduce these curvatures and rib hump. Many of these patients also have a number of psychological problems such as low self-esteem and self-image and occasionally pain. Cheryl would like to conduct a systematic review to find the evidence to underpin her practice.

Ten steps to help Cheryl develop the review question from her review topic

Cheryl starts developing her question by responding to the following ten steps.

1   Write down questions that have been in your mind from your area of practice.

Choose questions about which you are very curious and to which you would love to know the answer.

What are the effects of braces on the spinal curvature and rib hump?

What are patients' experiences of wearing a brace?

What are the positive effects of braces?

What are the negative effects of braces?

Are exercises for scoliosis effective?

Is surgery for treating scoliosis effective?

Is the practice of only observing and monitoring patients until they require surgery the best clinical practice?

2   Select one question that you would like to know the answer to.
     In patients with adolescent idiopathic scoliosis how effective is spinal bracing as
     compared with other treatments at reducing spinal curvature, rib hump and psy-
     chological problems?

3   Identify why it is interesting and worth investigating.
     If the brace is not effective at reducing the spinal curvature and rib hump, it may
     not be worth advising patients to use braces. It may also not be worth the sacri-
     fices that adolescents have to make to wear them.

4   Identify issues related to the question.
     Wearing a brace for 24 hours a day is not easy for teenagers. There are physical as
     well as psychological problems that need to be considered.

5   What will you gain by investigating the question?
     When the patients come for treatment I can be assured that they are not making
     the sacrifice of wearing a brace for nothing, but that the brace is really effective in
     treating the spine and rib hump.

6   What will your profession or other professions and service users gain?
     Both professionals and service users would be assured as to whether or not the
     treatment is an effective one. This would increase compliance and also has cost
     implications for health professionals.

7   What is the rationale for asking the question?
     I would like to be sure the treatment we are providing to these children is actually
     working and that there is an evidence base for its effectiveness.

8   Why does it excite you?
     It excites me because if the evidence is found to support the treatment effective-
     ness of bracing, then this may save a lot of young girls and boys the trauma of
     having spinal surgery in the future.

9   Is it a simple question or does it have several parts? If several parts, what are they?
     This question has three parts. The treatment has both physical effects and psycho-
     logical effects. The patients' and families' views are also very important.

10   In your opinion does the question address a significant problem? If so, answer the
     question 'So what?' here.
     Yes, it would address a significant problem, as identified earlier on; there is a lack
     of evidence supporting the use of bracing. It would provide the evidence to sup-
     port the judicious use of the brace in clinical practice.

Template to help you develop your review question from your review topic

Box 2.2 contains a template adapted from Bailey (1997) that you can use to help focus
your own research question.

   Once you have decided on a specific problem area and research question, the next
step is to refine and break down the research question and make it as comprehensive
and specific as possible. To do this you will need to consider the different categories
of research questions: not only are there background and foreground questions, but
also there are different types of foreground questions. Your review will differ based
on whether you are investigating the effectiveness of a treatment programme, seeking
to prevent a condition occurring, diagnosing a medical problem, looking at the cause

Box 2.2 Focusing the research question from the topic area

1   Write down three questions that have been in your mind from your area of practice. Choose questions about which you are very curious and to which you would love to know the answer.

2   Select one question that you would like to know the answer to.

3   Identify why it is interesting and worth investigating.

4   Identify issues related to the question.

5   What will you gain by investigating the question?

6   What will your profession or other professions and service users gain?

7   What is the rationale for asking the question?

8   Why does it excite you?

9   Is it a simple question or does it have several parts? If several parts, what are they?

10 In your opinion does the question address a significant problem? If so, answer the question 'So what?' here.

or prognosis of a specific condition or disease, or exploring patients', users' or nurses' perceptions and experiences.

Using background or foreground questions: what is the difference?

Background questions refer to general nursing questions about a patient. These can be research questions about their nursing/medical condition such as: what causes the condition or how is it treated? Is it a nursing intervention and/or clinical environmental related issue? Are patient safety and the quality of care an issue? The answers to these questions can be found in background sources such as textbooks or narrative reviews, which give an *overview* of the topic area.

Foreground questions answer a *specific* question about a specific topic. Foreground sources can be divided into primary sources such as original research articles published in peer-reviewed journals and secondary sources such as systematic reviews of the topic, and synopses and reviews of individual studies. Secondary sources are one step removed from the original research. Table 2.1 gives some examples of primary and secondary sources. The various concepts listed in the table will all be explained in this chapter.

Table 2.1 Types of studies in foreground sources

Primary sources – original research	Secondary sources – reviews of original research

• Experimental studies (an intervention is made)
   • Randomized controlled trial (RCT)
   • Controlled trials
 • Observational studies (no intervention or variables are manipulated)
   • Cohort studies
   • Case-control studies
   • Case reports/Case studies
 • Qualitative research studies
   • Phenomenological, ethnographic or grounded theory studies
	• Systematic reviews
	 • Systematic reviews with a meta-analysis
	 • Practice guidelines
	 • Decision analysis
	 • Consensus reports
	 • Editorial, commentary

Factors to consider when asking answerable and focused review questions

Blaikie (2007) suggests that the use of research or review questions is a neglected aspect in the design and conduct of research. He suggests that formulating a 'research question is the most critical and perhaps the most difficult part of any research design' (Blaikie 2007: 6). The formulation of the review question is crucial because the review question underpins all the aspects of the review methodology: every single step of the review is determined by the focused review question. The function of a review question can be summed up as follows:

• defines the nature and scope of the review

• identifies the keywords (together with the scoping search)

- determines the search strategy and the search to be undertaken
- provides guidance for selecting the primary research papers needed
- guides the data extraction and synthesis of the results.

When formulating a review question, it is important to ensure that you *ask an open question and not make a statement*. For example, rather than saying 'Braces improve the spinal curvatures of patients with scoliosis', as a novice student might, it would be preferable to ask, 'What effect do spinal braces have on patients with spinal curvatures?' In the first example you are making an assumption that braces will actually improve the back when they might not and they may even make the back worse. In this example you are making a statement and not asking a question. The first example is similar to a closed question and could introduce some bias (or errors). The second example is an open question and less biased. Asking this type of question will allow you to find research papers that discuss all the different effects of braces, both positive and negative. Another issue to consider is the way you word a question: it is best *to avoid questions that can be answered with a simple yes or no*. For example, asking. 'Do braces have an effect on the spinal curvatures of patients with spinal deformities?' can easily be answered with a yes or a no, whereas asking 'What effect do spinal braces have on patients with spinal curvatures?' encourages more discussion as well as being more open and unbiased. Table 2.2 lists some review questions to help you determine

Table 2.2 Main types of research questions

	Type	Description	Illustration
1	Treatment or therapy	Which treatment is most effective? Does it do more good than harm?	Is the use of dressing A better than dressing B in the treatment of venous leg ulcers?
2	Prevention	How to reduce the risk of disease	Do increasing levels of obesity increase the risk of developing diabetes?
3	Diagnosis	How to select and interpret diagnostic tests	Is having an x-ray as effective as having a computerized tomography (CT) scan for diagnosing a brain tumour?
4	Prognosis	How to anticipate the likely course of the disease	Are babies who are bottle fed more likely to be obese once they reach adulthood, compared with babies who are breastfed?
5	Causation	What are the risk factors for developing a certain condition?	Does exposure to parental alcohol during pregnancy increase the risk of foetal alcohol syndrome in newborn babies?
6	Patients' experiences and attitudes	How do people feel about this treatment or disease?	How do patients experience life with a venous leg ulcer?

what sort of evidence you are looking for within the primary research papers that you will select to answer your review question. One way to facilitate the development of your review question is to determine what kind of question you are asking (Flemming 1998). From there you can work out what kind of evidence you are looking for.

Examples of the main types of research questions

Some examples from practice can be found below:

1   Examples of treatment or therapy questions
   - What are the effects of braces on patients with spinal deformities?
   - How effective are antidepressive medications on anxiety and depression?
   - How effective are pressure-relieving mattresses at avoiding pressure sores?
   - Are hip protectors effective at avoiding fractures of the femur?

2   Examples of prevention questions
   - For patients of 70 years and older, how effective is the use of the influenza vaccine at preventing flu as compared with patients who have not received the vaccine?
   - How effective is school screening for scoliosis at reducing the risk of future surgery in patients with scoliosis?
   - How effective is intentional rounding in improving the quality of the patient experience?

3   Examples of diagnosis questions
   - In patients with suspected anorexia nervosa, what is the accuracy of a new scale compared with the 'gold standard' previously validated instrument?
   - In patients with suspected scoliosis (spinal curvature), what is the accuracy of a new non-invasive surface topography scanning device as compared with x-rays?

4   Examples of prognosis questions
   - How much more likely are babies who are bottle fed to catch colds than babies who are breastfed?
   - How much more likely are workers with musculoskeletal disorders to take sick leave as compared with workers diagnosed with stress?
   - How much more likely are children who are screened for scoliosis to have surgery than children who are not screened?

5   Examples of causation questions
   - For healthy post-menopausal patients on hormone replacement therapy (HRT), what are the increased risks for developing breast cancer?
   - In women taking oral contraceptives, is there an association between their use and breast cancer?
   - Does having a parent with a spinal deformity increase the risk of the child developing a scoliosis once they reach puberty?

6   Examples of patients' experiences and attitudes questions
   - What are teenagers' experiences of living with a spinal brace?
   - How do older patients experience life with cancer?
   - What are student nurses' experiences of life as a first-year university student?

Developing your review question further

If you have followed all of the steps above, you should by now have a tentative review question. In order to search for all the relevant papers on the topic, it is important that your question is both comprehensive and specific. It should include only one question and not two or three questions. A well-framed research question will have three or four elements (Flemming 1998). Once you have formulated your question the next step is to separate it into parts, as will be demonstrated in this section. The question formation usually includes identifying all the component parts, the population, the intervention, the comparative intervention (if any) and the outcomes that are measured. The acronym for this is PICO, which stands for population, intervention, comparative intervention and outcome. PICO is designed mainly for questions of therapeutic interventions (Khan et al. 2003). Another useful acronym is PEO, which stands for patient, exposure and outcome. PEO is used most frequently for qualitative questions (Khan et al. 2003). A good way to identify the different parts of your question for PICO formats is to make a table containing four rows, one for each letter of the acronym. Table 2.3 shows what type of information to include in each of the sections. Table 2.4 shows some completed examples. For qualitative questions that use the PEO format you will need to create a table containing three rows. Table 2.5 shows you what to include in each of the sections.

Table 2.3 Component parts to consider when asking clear focused review questions

P Population and their problem	Here you need to state the clinical diagnosis or disease, the age, gender and any other relevant factors related to the population you would like to include. The population group needs to be specified whatever type of question you are considering.
I Intervention or exposure	If you are planning to evaluate a specific intervention you will need to state the type of intervention that you are seeking to evaluate, such as the type of drug and any specifics related to it like dosage and other relevant factors. If you are not looking at an intervention but are considering a specific 'exposure' (this term is used loosely) such as 'witnessed resuscitation' or 'domestic violence', you should use the E as in the PEO acronym instead of the PICO acronym. The exposure component can also be regarded as an 'issue' that the patients or the population you are considering including in your review have undergone.
C Comparative intervention	In a therapeutic question you will usually have a comparator (even if it is standard care). It is also possible to look at interventions without including a comparative intervention. For qualitative review questions or those involving a specific exposure or issue, this component is usually left out.
O Outcomes or themes	When writing down your outcomes, you need to consider the factors or issues you are looking for or measuring. For example, are you looking for any improvements in pain or mobility, or any other outcomes? With qualitative studies these will usually be the patients' and/or the nurse 'healthcare worker' experiences.

In Tables 2.4 and 2.5 you can find some examples of using both the PICO and the PEO acronyms to formulate your own questions. The PICO questions are usually quantitative questions and the PEO ones are usually qualitative questions.

Table 2.4 Examples of using PICO to ask clear quantitative questions

	Example 1	Example 2	Example 3	Example 4
P Population and their problem	In patients with acute asthma	In children with a spinal deformity	In children with a fever	Among family members of patients with mental health problems
I Intervention or issue	how effective are antibiotics	how effective is bracing	how effective is paracetamol as compared with	how effective is listening to tranquil music, or audiotaped comedy routines
C Comparative intervention	as compared with standard care	as compared with observation	ibuprofen	as compared with standard care (none)
O Outcomes or themes	at reducing sputum production and coughing?	at reducing the scoliosis curvature?	at reducing fever and infection?	in reducing reported anxiety?

Table 2.5 Examples of using PEO to ask clear qualitative questions

	Example 1	Example 2	Example 3	Example 4
P Population and their problem	In teenagers with a spinal deformity	Older patients with cancer	Student nurses in their first year at university	Family members of patients with mental health problems
E Exposure	the development of a spinal deformity	cancer	studying to be a nurse at university and in their first year	having a family member with mental health problem
O Outcomes or themes	the patients' views	the patients' views	the students' views	the patients' views

Regarding Cheryl's question from the case study, the structured question can be broken down into the component parts as defined by the PICO framework as follows:

- In patients with adolescent idiopathic scoliosis (P)
- how effective is spinal bracing (I)
- as compared with observation (C)
- at reducing spinal curvature, rib hump and psychological problems (O)?

Table 2.6 shows how to separate the component parts of Cheryl's question using the PICO method.

Table 2.6 Cheryl's question broken down using the PICO method

P	I	C	O
Patients with adolescent idiopathic scoliosis	how effective is spinal bracing	as compared with other treatments	at reducing spinal curvature, rib hump and psychological problems?

Cheryl's nursing colleague Kirsty, who works in the same spinal unit, is more interested in the patients' views. Kirsty's question is 'What are the lived experiences of patients with adolescent idiopathic scoliosis of having scoliosis and wearing a brace?' Table 2.7 shows how Kirsty's question would be separated into its component parts using the PEO method.

Table 2.7 Kirsty's question broken down using the PEO method

P	E	O
Patients with adolescent idiopathic scoliosis	having scoliosis and wearing a brace	lived experiences of having scoliosis and wearing a brace

Practice session 2.1

Now we have seen how to split different types of questions into their component parts, why don't you try to split your own question? Use the templates provided in Boxes 2.3 and 2.4 to divide your intervention or exposure question into PICO or PEO. If your question has more than one population group, please adapt the template as appropriate.

Box 2.3   Template for splitting a quantitative intervention question into PICO component parts

P	I	C	O

Box 2.4 Template for splitting a qualitative experience question into PEO component parts		
P	E	O

Relating your question to the research design: what types of study designs should you look for to answer your research question?

Now that you have split your question into its component parts, the next step is to think about how your question relates to the research design of the studies that you plan to include within your review and which will form the basis for answering your review question. Why do we need this? Once you have formulated your question you will need to search for papers that answer your question. Khan et al. (2003) recommend the inclusion of the study designs of the proposed studies while still in the process of formulating your review question. So rather than using PICO or PEO you could adapt this to use PICOT or PEOT, where the T stands for the *type* of study or research design.

The type of research design can be thought of as the structure of the research study. It is a whole plan of how all the parts of the project fit together, including who the subjects are, what instruments were used if any, how the study was conducted and analysed and finally discussed.

Types of research designs

Some of the common quantitative and qualitative research designs are described below.

Types of quantitative designs

Case report, case study, case series

A case report is a report of a treatment of an individual patient. Case reports are generally undertaken and reported when a patient of particular interest or with special or complex characteristics is treated by a nurse. For example, you may come across a patient who has a condition that you have never seen or heard of before and you are uncertain what to do. A search for case series or case reports may reveal information that will help you treat your patient. When the first case of Creutzfeldt-Jakob disease

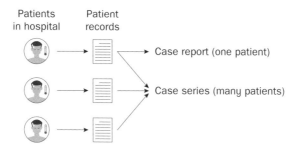

Figure 2.2 A schematic for a case report and case series.

(CJD) was treated, it would have been reported as a case study. When a few cases are reported, this becomes a case series. Figure 2.2 illustrates the design of a case report study, with the schematic for a case report and case series research design.

Case–control studies

Case–control studies are research studies in which patients who already have a specific condition are compared with people who do not. They rely on medical records and patient recall for data collection. In other words they are retrospective studies (looking back) that can be done fairly quickly by taking the patients' histories. A good example of this can be seen by considering the time during the acquired immune deficiency syndrome (AIDS) epidemic when case–control studies identified not only risk groups such as homosexual men, intravenous drug users and blood transfusion recipients but also risk factors, such as having multiple sex partners and not using condoms. Based on such studies, blood banks restricted high-risk individuals from donating blood, and educational programmes began to promote safer behaviours. As a result of these precautions, the speed of transmission of the human immunodeficiency virus (HIV) was greatly reduced, even before the virus had been identified (Schulz and Grimes 2002: 431). The schematic for a case–control research design can be seen in Figure 2.3.

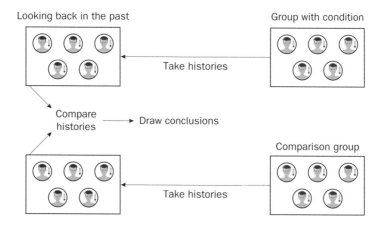

Figure 2.3 A schematic for a case–control research design.

Cohort studies

Cohort studies are usually made up of a large population. The cohort study design follows patients who have a specific condition or who receive a particular treatment over time. These patients are compared with another group that has not been affected by the condition or treatment. For example, you may be interested in the long-term effects on nurses who smoke. In a cohort study you would follow-up a group of nurses who smoke and a group who do not smoke and then compare their outcomes over time. One of the main problems with this design is that they can take a very long time to conduct. If you started following both groups of nurses when they were in their twenties and measured the outcomes every 10 years until they retired, this would mean the study would take over 40 years to complete. The schematic for a cohort research design can be seen in Figure 2.4.

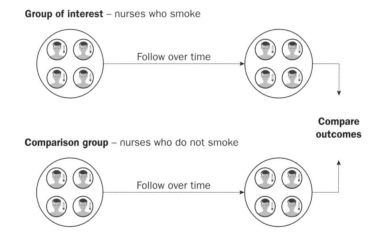

Figure 2.4 A schematic for a cohort research design.

Randomized controlled trials

Randomized controlled trials study the effect of treatments such as therapy, medication or programmes on real patients. The methods they include try to reduce the potential for bias and the patients may be randomly assigned into a treated group and a control group. The inclusion of the control group, who have exactly the same conditions as the treated group with the exception of the treatment itself, allows us to ensure that it was the treatment itself that had an effect on the patients and not anything else. A schematic for an RCT research design can be seen in Figure 2.5.

Systematic reviews

As discussed in Chapter 1, an extensive literature search is conducted that uses only studies with sound methodology. The studies are collected, reviewed and assessed, data are extracted and the results summarized according to predetermined criteria of the review question (Figure 2.6).

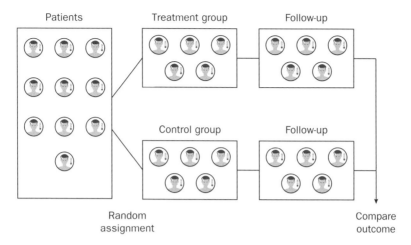

Figure 2.5 A schematic for a randomized control trial research design.

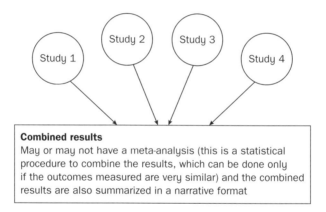

Figure 2.6 An illustration of how several studies can be combined to produce a definitive result.

Meta-analysis

A meta-analysis is a statistical procedure that is used in some systematic reviews. A meta-analysis examines a group of valid quantitative studies on a topic and combines the results using accepted statistical methodology to reach a consensus on the overall results. A meta-analysis can be used only on studies where the research papers included are very similar and where the outcome measures of the included research papers are the same. Only a small proportion of systematic reviews include a meta-analysis.

Types of qualitative research designs

The three most common types of qualitative research designs are described below.

Phenomenological research design

When nurses apply a phenomenological research design, they are concerned with the lived experiences of people (Greene 1997). This could be the lived experiences of patients with a particular condition, the experiences of older nurses, or the experiences of nursing students while training in hospitals.

Ethnographic research design

An ethnographic research design was originally used by anthropologists who went to live with native peoples in remote places in order to understand how they lived. According to Spradley (1979), ethnography is 'the work of describing a culture' and the goal of ethnographic research is 'to understand another way of life from the native point of view' (Spradley 1979: 3). Within nursing practice, the term 'native' is used loosely and can refer to different nursing cultures that can be found within mental health nursing as compared with adult and paediatric nursing. Spradley (1979: iv) suggests that ethnography is a useful tool for 'understanding how other people see their experience'. He emphasizes, however, that 'rather than *studying people*, ethnography means *learning from people*' (Spradley 1979: 3, our emphases). If we apply this in a nursing context, we may be interested in learning from nurses who work in a specific culture or area, such as mental health nurses who work in prisons, nurses who work in an intensive care unit or nurses who work in palliative care. Similarly, the research may focus on the lived experience of patients/carers who have stayed within these clinical environments and settings.

Grounded theory research design

The grounded theory research design was developed by Glaser and Strauss (1967). This method is used as both a qualitative research method and a method of data analysis. In grounded theory the researcher aims to develop a theory that can explain events and behaviour, giving predictions and control over a situation. Grounded theory is a research method that operates almost in a reverse fashion from traditional research and at first may appear to be in contradiction to the scientific method. Rather than beginning with a hypothesis, the first step is data collection, through a variety of methods. From the data collected, the key points are marked with a series of themes or codes, which are extracted from the text. The codes or themes are grouped into similar *concepts* in order to make them more workable. From these concepts, *categories* are formed, which are the basis for the creation of a *theory*, or a reverse engineered hypothesis. This contradicts the traditional model of research, where the researcher chooses a theoretical framework, and only then applies this model to the phenomenon to be studied (Glaser and Strauss 1967).

Relating a specific research question to an appropriate research design

Having discussed the main types of quantitative and qualitative research designs, how does the specific type of research question relate to the appropriate research design? A summary of the types of research designs best suited to the different types of review questions can be found in Table 2.8.

Table 2.8 Summary of the types of research designs best suited to the different types of review questions

Type of question	Suggested best type of study			
	Least biased ——————————————————— Most biased			
Treatment or therapy	RCT >	cohort >	case–control >	case series
Diagnosis	Retrospective, blind comparison with gold standard			
Aetiology or harm	RCT >	cohort >	case–control >	case series
Prognosis		cohort >	case–control >	case series
Prevention	RCT >	cohort >	case–control >	case series
Experiences or perceptions	Qualitative studies: most common are phenomenological, ethnographic and grounded theory			

Questions of therapy, causes and prevention that can best be answered by RCT can also be answered by meta-analysis and systematic reviews.
Qualitative questions where a significant amount of research on the same research question has been conducted can also be answered by systematic reviews.

Key points

- Selecting a topic area for your systematic review is the first step towards undertaking the review.
- The specific topic you select may arise from a number of different triggers.
- Once you have selected your research topic, the next step is to narrow this down to a specific research question.
- There are two main types of questions: background questions that are general nursing questions and foreground questions that answer a specific question about a specific topic.
- Foreground questions and sources can be divided into primary sources such as original research and secondary sources such as systematic reviews.
- Formulating research questions is the most critical and perhaps the most difficult part of any research design.
- The research question underpins all the components of the review methods.
- It is important to ensure that you ask an open question.
- It is best to avoid closed questions that can be answered with a simple yes or no.
- The main types of research questions relate to treatment or therapy, prevention, diagnosis, prognosis, causation and experiences.
- It is important that your question is both comprehensive and specific.
- A well-framed research question will have three or four elements.

- The question formation usually includes identifying all the component parts: the population, the intervention or exposure, the comparative intervention (if any) and the outcomes that are measured. The acronyms for these are PICO or PEO.
- It is important to match your question to the appropriate research design.
- The research design can be thought of as the structure of the research study.

Summary

This chapter discussed the different ways of finding topic areas for your review and described the meaning and functions of an answerable and focused review question. The chapter presented the main types of focused research questions together with some examples from nursing practice. The chapter discussed the different types of research questions and the importance of selecting the appropriate research design for the type of research question you have selected. A number of templates were provided to help you formulate your own answerable and focused systematic review question.

Questions and Answers (Q&A)

(Q) Are there any ways to support you in identifying an area to focus a research question?

(A) An effective way of identifying an area to focus your research question is to look at what is topical in the nursing press. For example, the High Impact Actions for Nursing and Midwifery: The Essential Collection (NHS Institute for Innovation and Improvement 2010) offers some key areas that may help you to focus your research. Similarly, looking at the news headlines in specific journals may help you generate and focus your ideas. Finally, talking to colleagues in practice is a great way of identifying areas to focus a research question.

(Q) Why is it important to develop the correct research question?

(A) Investing the time and effort to develop a sound research question will result in a more robust systematic review. For example, ensuring you have the best designs/drawings/plans for building a new house will ensure the foundations and building is strong and long-lasting. Similarly, by having a robust research question, your results and findings will be reliable.

3
Creating the protocol for your systematic review

Overview

- The importance of writing a protocol for your review
- Steps to take when planning your review
- Sections to include within your protocol
- Brief overview of all the steps/sections to include within your protocol

The importance of writing a protocol for your review

Writing a protocol of what you intend to include before you start your systematic review is very important. A protocol (also called a 'plan') describes in advance the review question and your rationale for the proposed methods you will use. It also includes details of how different types of studies will be located, appraised and synthesized (Petticrew and Roberts 2006). Describing your methods in advance is a way of trying to minimize bias (something that causes a consistent deviation from the truth) as you cannot start changing the way you review the papers once you see the results of the identified studies. For instance, if you said in the protocol that you will be including only RCTs and then found a study by a well-known nurse or healthcare professional which was not an RCT, the temptation might be for you to include it. However, you would not be able to do this as you have stated otherwise in your protocol. Another important reason to undertake a protocol for your review is that you can then show this to other colleagues you work with, patients with the specific problem and/or your supervisor. They can read your protocol and provide you with further suggestions to improve it, as you may not have thought of relevant issues that are important to the patients, service users and other nurses and healthcare professionals.

Although most nurses who are conducting their first review will conduct it on their own, the highest quality systematic reviews, such as those undertaken by the Cochrane Centre, Campbell Collaboration and the Joanna Briggs Institute, are usually undertaken in teams. Conducting a review in a team decreases bias and increases the validity (or truthfulness) of the results. If you are a student nurse or a clinician without access to a team, it is perfectly acceptable to conduct a review on your own, so long as you acknowledge that doing so may decrease the validity of your results and increase the level of bias in your study.

Practical Tip

If you are undertaking a systematic review on your own before preparing the protocol, always talk to other professional colleagues and academic supervisors in your area about your proposed idea and reasons for the systematic review. This approach will help you formulate your ideas and enrich the protocol, which is essentially the blueprint for the systematic review.

Steps to take when planning your review

Once you have formulated your review question, it is a good idea to undertake a quick general search (also called a scoping search) to make sure that there are no systematic literature reviews already available or in progress that have already addressed your review question. Box 3.1 shows some common websites where you can check this out (please note that this list is not exhaustive). An excellent checklist is in a book called *Systematic Reviews* available for free on the Centre for Reviews and Dissemination website (see below).

Box 3.1   Websites for checking for systematic literature reviews

- Cochrane Centre and Library:
  www.uk.cochrane.org
- TRIP database:
  www.tripdatabase.com
- Centre for Reviews and Dissemination (University of York):
  www.york.ac.uk/inst/crd
- Campbell Collaboration:
  www.campbellcollaboration.org
- Cochrane Qualitative Research Methods Group:
  http://qim.cochrane.org/
- Cumulative Index of Nursing and Allied Health Literature (CINAHL):
  https://www.ebscohost.com/academic/cinahl-plus-with-full-text
- Worldviews on Evidence-Based Nursing:
  http://onlinelibrary.wiley.com/journal/10.1111/(ISSN)1741-6787
- Evidence-Based Nursing:
  http://ebn.bmj.com/
- The JBI database of systematic reviews and implementation reports:
  http://joannabriggslibrary.org/

If you find a narrative review that was published recently, it is fine to go ahead with your systematic literature review, because a systematic review is considered to be a much higher quality review. If you find a systematic literature review exactly like the one your protocol aims to carry out, there are a number of strategies you can follow; for example, you can look to see if the review you found in your preliminary search was conducted recently or a number of years previously. If a number of papers have been published since the last systematic review, it is still fine to go ahead with your own systematic review as your review will contribute new knowledge. If no new papers have been published since the last systematic review, there is no point in conducting a review that would produce exactly the same results. The best thing to do in this case is to change or 'tweak' the population group, the intervention or the outcomes, so your specific review question will be slightly different from the previously published systematic review. For example, in Cheryl's case, her title is 'In patients with adolescent idiopathic scoliosis how effective is spinal bracing as compared with other treatments at reducing spinal curvature, rib hump and psychological problems?' If she found a systematic literature review that had already been conducted and no new papers had been published since, she could change the population group and look at adults. Alternatively she could look at a subgroup of the population, such as obese adolescents or change the intervention, comparative group or specific outcomes to be investigated.

Practice session 3.1

For your own review question, search the websites above to identify whether your research question has already been addressed through a systematic review.

Sections to include within your protocol

The length of time you devote to writing up your protocol depends on the specific circumstances in which you are writing your review. If you are writing up the review to answer a research question for yourself, it is acceptable for the protocol of your review to be quite brief and sketchy. If you are proposing a protocol for a more formal review, for instance if you are conducting this review as part of your continuing professional development, or if it is a requirement for a module on a formal undergraduate or postgraduate nursing programme, such as a dissertation, the protocol of your review will need to be more detailed and precise.

Practical Tip

Investing the time and effort to devise a sound protocol at this early stage will only serve to enhance the quality and outcomes of your systematic review.

The sections within the protocol and in the full review are identical, except that in the protocol, the sections are quite brief and will not include the results and discussion sections of the review. Once you have written your protocol and are completing the full review, you will need to go over each section in more detail and include your results and discussion sections as well.

A brief overview of all the sections to include within your protocol (and later your full review) is listed below. Chapters 4–12 provide a much more detailed discussion of the full process to conduct each section of the review. Full details for undertaking each part of the review can be found in the chapter indicated.

Brief overview of all the steps/sections to include within your protocol

Step 1: Developing an answerable review question (Chapter 2)

Step 2: Writing the background to your review (briefly) (Chapter 4)

Step 3: Writing the objectives (or purpose of the review) (Chapter 5)

Step 4: Specifying your inclusion and exclusion criteria (Chapter 5)

Step 5: Conducting the search strategy (Chapter 6)

Step 6: Selecting, appraising and extracting the relevant data from your research papers to answer your review question (Chapter 7–9)

Step 7: Plans for synthesizing the data (Chapter 10)

Developing a review question has already been discussed in Chapter 2. The background section is discussed in the next chapter (4) and the remaining steps will be discussed in Chapters 5–10. A brief summary of what should be included in each step or section of your review protocol is found below.

Step 1: Developing an answerable review question (Chapter 2)

Already discussed in Chapter 2.

Step 2: Writing the background to your review (briefly) (Chapter 4)

The background section of a systematic review is similar to writing a narrative review. The purpose of the background section is to provide an overview of the specific area of the review, highlight the clinical problems associated with the area or question, discuss the relevant reviews within the specific clinical area and clarify the gap in systematic reviews in this area.

Step 3: Writing the objectives (or purpose of the review) (Chapter 5)

The purpose of writing out the objectives of your review is to clarify your reason for conducting the review. If we go back to the review on braces, we defined our objective as follows: 'The purpose of our review was to evaluate the effectiveness of braces on patients with spinal curvature and rib hump'.

Step 4: Specifying your inclusion and exclusion criteria (Chapter 5)

In this section you need to decide on the specific criteria by which your protocol aims to select (or not select) the primary papers for your review. These will include specific criteria on the types of subjects, interventions (or exposure), comparative group and outcomes, as well as the types of studies to include in the protocol and subsequent review.

Step 5: Conducting the search strategy (Chapter 6)

The search strategy describes how and where your protocol relates to searching for your primary research papers to include for your review. To ensure that your search strategy is replicable, it is important to include a detailed description of your search strategy that is based on your review question.

Step 6: Selecting, appraising and extracting the relevant data from your research papers to answer your review question (Chapter 7–9)

In this section you need to describe the process of how your protocol will aid you in selecting your papers, how your protocol aims to evaluate your papers, what framework you will be using to do this, and finally the process of extracting data from your papers to answer the review question. In other words you will be explaining in detail how your protocol will help you to go through your papers and take out the relevant information to answer your review question. For example, if you were interested in looking at the effectiveness of the Weight Watchers diet or eating programme, you would want to know the weight of the participants in all your papers before they started on Weight Watchers, as well as after finishing the programme. You would read through all your research papers to find the figures that address this and 'extract' them. Full details of how to do this are given in Chapters 7–9.

Step 7: Plans for synthesizing the data (Chapter 10)

In this step of the protocol it is important to describe the methods that you plan to use to synthesize your data (both the qualitative as well as the quantitative data if you are conducting a mixed methods systematic review)

Below we have included an example of a real student's systematic review dissertation following feedback from readers so that you can see for yourself what a protocol may look like. Please note that although the content of the example protocol may now be dated and the rules and regulations mentioned within this example may now have changed, we would like you to concentrate mainly on the *format* and not so much on the example below. Please note that the student gave their permission for their work to be used as an example.

Fay: Example of a student's protocol

Included in this section is an example of a full protocol developed by a student, Fay (not her real name), who has kindly given permission to illustrate what a protocol looks like. Fay was studying for a Bachelor of Science (BSc) in Nursing. The authors acknowledge that the protocol was developed a number of years ago. This protocol is only intended to illustrate how a protocol can be developed and may therefore not be reflective of current policy and practice. The area of interest of the student conducting this systematic review was 'urinary tract infections (UTI)' and the aim of her review was to evaluate the existing guidelines that promote the practice of not using antiseptics at catheter insertion. So her research question was '*In patients requiring urinary catherisation, is sterile catheter insertion more effective than non-sterile insertion at reducing the incidence of catheter associated urinary tract infection (CAUTI)?*'

 Step 1: Developing an answerable review question/title (Chapter 2)

Example: Fay's protocol

Title: In patients requiring urinary catheterisation, is sterile catheter insertion more effective than non-sterile insertion at reducing the incidence of catheter associated urinary tract infection (CAUTI)?

(Title page for protocol)

Step 2: Background

Urinary catheterisation of patients is a common nursing procedure used both in the hospital and in the community. According to Dougherty and Lister (2004, pg 333) catheter associated infections are the most common nosocomial infection, counting up to around 45% of all hospital acquired infections. Hospital acquired infection can be defined as an infection that is neither present, nor incubating, at the time of admission to hospital (Hospital Acquired Infection [online]). Studies by Bryan and Reynolds (1984, pg 494–498) and Turck and Stamm (1981, pg 651–654) concluded that between 75% and 80% of all healthcare associated UTIs follow the insertion of a urinary catheter and a study by Glynn et al (1997) which investigated 40 English hospitals, estimated that around 26% of all hospitalised patients have a urinary catheter inserted, whilst Parker (1999, pg 563–574) and Godfrey and Evans (2000, pg 682–690) suggest that 4% of patients in the community, at some point, will have a catheter inserted. Furthermore, complications that may arise from urinary catheterisation include structural damage to the urinary tract, bleeding, false passage, and urinary tract infections and bacteriuria (Joanna Briggs). It is estimated that CAUTI costs the National Health Service (NHS) £1,327 per patient and because it increases the period of hospitalisation of such patients, by approximately three to six days, costs approximately increase by £124 million per year (Hart, 2008, pg 44–48; SSHAIP, 2004, [online]).

Catheterisation – types and indications

A catheter is a tubular device which is passed through the urethra into the bladder in order to drain urine or to instill medical treatment (Dougherty and Lister, 2004, pg 330–333; Steward, in BJN monograph, 2001, pg 42). Catheterisation is indicated in and used to relieve obstructed flow of urine, to measure the residual amount in the bladder, to provide post-operative drainage following bladder, vaginal and prostate surgery, in monitoring hourly urine output in the critically ill patient, and in continence care (Brunner and Suddarth, 1992, pg 682; Steward, in BJN monograph, 2001, pg 42). Insertion of a urinary catheter is a common procedure in both acute and primary care settings, and careful consideration is always required over the need for, versus, the risk of this procedure. Urethral catheterisation may be performed as an indwelling or an intermittent procedure. Indwelling catheterisation consists of continuous catheter drainage which can be sub-classified into short term (1–7 days), mid-term (7–28 days) and long term (28 days up to 3 months) (Hart, 2008, pg 44–48; Head, 2006, pg 33–36; RCN, 2008, pg 2–55).

   Intermittent catheterisation consists of episodic introduction of a catheter into the bladder to drain urine out (Dougherty and Lister, 2004, pg 335). The catheter is passed via the urethra and removed soon after the bladder urine is drained. In recent years this technique has become noticeably popular, and can be carried out by the patient him/herself or by the nurse. This form of catheterisation is indicated for the drainage of a poorly functioning bladder (as is found in spinal cord injury patients and those with neurological disorders) and for urinary drainage in the peri-operative period. Its main advantage is that the patient is left catheter-free in between catheterisations (Dougherty and Lister, 2004, pg 335; Robinson, 2007, pg 48–56). Intermittent catheterisation is also commonly used to instill medications, measure residual urine, and it is also used to instill contrast material into the bladder to study the bladder and the urethra (Hart, 2008, pg 44–48). Lapides et al (2002, pg 1584–1586) and Wilson (1998, pg S10–13) advocate that this procedure should be undertaken as a sterile procedure in the hospital environment due to the high risk of hospital acquired infections, while in the community a clean technique should be used.

Catheter associated urinary tract infection (CAUTI)

Catheters are a major cause of urinary tract infection; they pave the way for micro-organisms to enter the bladder. Since they are a foreign body they consequently offer a surface for micro-organisms to grow on and act as a route for micro-organisms to gain access into the urinary tract. Insertion may result in physical damage to the urethra and catheters may interfere with the body's immune responses and may cause a chemical induced inflammation in the urethral and bladder mucosa (Walsh, 1997, pg 672). All these factors are responsible at predisposing to CAUTI.

Catheter associated urinary tract infections may affect any part of the urinary system and are caused by exogenous micro-organisms or endogenous faecal or urethral micro-organisms (Godfrey and Evans, 2000, pg 682–690). Saint and Lipsky (1999, pg 800–808) suggest that these infections can also be acquired by cross-contamination from other patients or hospital health care workers or by exposure to contaminated solutions or non-sterile equipment. The normal urinary tract is least sterile near the urethral orifice; hence, micro-organisms can inhabit the meatus or distal urethra, and thus, can be introduced directly into the bladder on catheter insertion (Parker, 1999, pg 563–574).

In long term indwelling catheterisation micro-organisms may enter the urinary tract through two possible routes, from the catheter lumen (intraluminal infection) or via the space between the walls of the catheter and the urethra (the periurethral or extraluminal route) (Getliffe, 1996, pg 548–554). Therefore shorter periods of catheterisation and minimal catheter and drainage bag handling are recognised forms of preventing such infections (Mangnall and Waterson, 2006, pg 49–56). Alexander et al (2000, pg 319) indicate that urinary infections are most common in females. The female urethra is shorter and its external meatus is closer to the perineal area and thus offers a shorter distance for microbes to reach the urinary tract (Tambyah, 2004, pg S44–S48).

CAUTI is asymptomatic in the majority of cases (Tambyah et al, 2000, pg 678–682); however, Godfrey and Evans (2000, pg 682–690) clarify that CAUTI can present with signs and symptoms such as: pyrexia, pyuria, urinary bypassing of the catheter, cloudy foul-smelling urine, confusion in elderly patients, haematuria and back pain. These symptoms may vary with the age and sex of the patient and also with the severity and site of the infection. Pickerman (1994, pg 66–68) suggests that these signs and symptoms occur when the bacteria invade the bladder mucosa resulting in inflammation. Diagnosis is established after obtaining a urine sample for culture and sensitivity. A bacterial count of 100,000 organisms (or CFU) per millilitre is considered to be significant of urinary tract infection. Bacteriuria and urinary tract infection are two terms used interchangeably in the nursing literature. Bacteriuria is the presence of bacteria in the urine; however, according to Higgins (1995, pg 33–35) bacteriuria in patients with indwelling and intermittent catheters does not always suggest a diagnosis of urinary tract infection (UTI).

Guidelines on catheterisation technique

Guidelines by both the Royal College of Nurses (RCN, 2008, pg 42–45) and the National Institute for Health and Clinical Excellence (NIHCE, 2003, pg 8–11) emphasise the use of aseptic technique at catheter insertion in order to prevent catheter associated urinary tract infection. This recommended aseptic technique is mainly a non-touch procedure which involves preparation of the environment and equipment, and hand washing which is considered to be most effective at reducing the risk of hospital acquired infection (DoH, 2001, pg S21–37; Gould et al, 2007, pg 109–115). It also involves the use of sterile gloves and disposable aprons; Callaghan (1998, pg 37–420) points out that disposable aprons are worn to protect nurses' clothing from contamination, and thus, reduce the risk of transferring micro-organisms to other patients. The NMC (2008) suggests cleaning of the meatal area with sterile agents and use of sterile lubricating gel in order to make catheterisation more comfortable and reduce the risk of urethral trauma. However, Dougherty and Lister (2004, pg 333–334) consider vigorous meatal cleaning as unnecessary; on the other hand, Tambyah et al (1999, pg 131–136) emphasise that infection occurs extraluminally on catheter insertion, and thus, suggest that antiseptic cleaning of the meatus is vital. Leaver (2007, pg 39–42) also states that meatal cleansing mechanically removes exudates and smegma.

Rationale of the study

Opinions as to the choice of meatal cleansing solution (whether it is an antiseptic or a simple sterile solution) and how sterile the whole procedure of catheter insertion should be have varied over time and from region to region. Other National guidelines found in documents such as Winning Ways (DH 2003) and Essential Steps to Safe, Clean Care (DH 2006) are aimed at reducing risks of and the incidence of health care associated infections (HCAI). These documents are based on the NIHCE guidelines (2003) which in turn have been based on EPIC guidelines developed by Pratt et al (2001). The latter guidelines were updated in EPIC 2 which was published in 2006. Although such publications strive to present clear information on what needs to be done in specific situations to reduce risks it seems that they may remain open to interpretation if they are not based on solid reliable evidence. EPIC's (Pratt et al, 2006, pg S30) recommendations on cleaning the urethral meatus using sterile normal saline and using sterile non-antiseptic lubricating gel were, as admitted by the authors, based on expert opinion. It is no wonder, therefore, that the type of cleansing solution to be used is not even mentioned in the RCN guidelines (RCN, 2008), and the NIHCE guidelines (2003) leave the choice of cleansing solution to the health carer and recommend adherence to local guidelines and policies. Pellowe (2004, pg 13–14) suggests that detailed operational protocols at local level, must incorporate such guidelines and principles for preventing HCAI's such as CAUTI. Furthermore, as evidenced by comments in a letter to the editor (Panknin and Althaus, 2001, pg 146–147) that criticises EPIC's decision on including their recommendation on meatal cleansing when it was based only on expert opinion, the opinion in other countries in Europe regarding disinfection of the meatal area disagrees with guidelines in this country. The authors of this letter claim that antiseptic disinfection is the norm in their institution and in their opinion it explains their lower incidence of CAUTI.

The objective of this study, hence, is to identify the relevant literature that exists that could serve as evidence that would settle this discrepancy in opinion. Three systematic reviews were identified in the literature. The review by Jamison et al (2004) focuses mainly on the use of catheter types in management of the neurogenic bladder whereas the review by Niel-Weise and van den Broek (2005) looked at studies comparing urethral indwelling, intermittent and supra-pubic catheterisation. The review by Lockwood et al (2004, pg 271–291) treated the issue of sterility at insertion very briefly; only two relevant studies were included. Since these reviews focused mainly on other catheter related matters, their search strategy, therefore, could have resulted in studies relevant to the antiseptic issue being missed and left out. This study focused solely on this particular issue of sterility at catheter insertion and adopted a search strategy that would include as many of the studies that specifically dealt with this topic.

 ## Step 3: Objectives

The aim of this review was to establish whether urinary catheterisation performed using a strict sterile technique is more effective than a non-sterile insertion technique at reducing the incidence of CAUTI in patients requiring urinary catheterisation. Evidence from studies dealing with sterile/non-sterile insertion technique and more specifically the steps involved in it (i.e. antiseptic periurethral cleaning, hand washing and sterile gloves, and sterile or antiseptic containing lubricating gel) have been evaluated.

 ## Step 4: Criteria for considering studies for this review

Introduction

The criteria for the selection of studies to be included in a review need to be defined ahead of the selection process in order to avoid selection bias (Khan et al 2003, pg 29). The components of the structured question are used to generate a list of selection criteria. Using the PICO (Population, Intervention, Comparison and Outcome) framework facilitates the process. The study types or designs are identified after considering their likely suitability at answering the review question and their level on the evidence hierarchy, while also bearing in mind the probable abundance or sparsity of the relevant studies. Torgerson (2003, pg 27–28) recommends a rapid scope of the literature early in the planning stage to establish how plentiful relevant studies are; this also serves to identify existing reviews, however, Torgerson also warns that this could be a source of bias in the review

Types of studies

The best study designs to answer review questions regarding effectiveness of an intervention are comparative studies; these studies compare the effect of the intervention on outcome in the study group with outcome in the control group (who are not exposed to the intervention being assessed). Such studies feature high on the hierarchy of evidence when allocation to the two groups is randomised and concealed, the randomised controlled trials (RCTs); bias is avoided since any confounding varia- bles are equally distributed between the two groups (Craig and Smyth 2002, pg 89–92). However, following a rapid scope of the literature, it was evident that studies relevant to the review question were unlikely to be numerous; therefore it was deemed neces- sary that other designs (shown in Table 3.1) that are not considered as sound as RCTs, were also included.

The participants

Patients who required and underwent urinary catheterisation, whether indwelling (short term or long term) or intermittent, and which was performed by a healthcarer were included in the review. However, patients who underwent intermittent self-catheterisation were excluded along with those having pre-existing urinary tract infections, those who had undergone urological surgery and those who were on antibiotics.

Types of intervention

The interventions under investigation were the sterile or aseptic catheter insertion technique and the specific steps involved in the process namely hand washing, sterile gloves and gowns, antiseptic meatal cleansing and use of antiseptic lubricating gel.

Types of comparison

Non-sterile or clean catheter insertion techniques were the comparisons or controls examined; these included insertion techniques or their component steps that did not use antiseptics or sterile equipment as is used in the sterile technique. Also included were insertion techniques where one or more of the specific steps of the sterile approach were either omitted or modified and/or where any of the following occurred:

- Hand washing is omitted or modified and/or
- no sterile gloves are used and/or
- no sterile gowns are used and/or
- no antiseptic meatal cleansing and/or
- lubricating gel used contains no antiseptic.

Types of outcome measures

The rate of incidence of CAUTI was considered as the outcome measure. CAUTI was identified as established by the presence of its clinical symptoms and/or the presence of significant bacteriuria. Significant bacteriuria was defined as 100,000 CFU/ml and was considered to be more reliable at diagnosing CAUTI since the latter may be asymptomatic. It was assumed that CAUTI that could, safely, be attributed directly to catheter insertion would occur within the first few days following insertion and hence urine samples showing significant bacteriuria within this period would be most reliable.

Inclusion/exclusion criteria

A summary of the inclusion/exclusion criteria can be seen in Table 3.1.

 Table 3.1 Inclusion and exclusion criteria

	Inclusion criteria	Exclusion criteria
Population	Male or female patients undergoing urinary catheterisation performed by healthcarers Short term/long term indwelling or intermittent catheterisation Setting: hospital, rehabilitation unit or nursing home	Intermittent self-catheterisation, supra-pubic catheterisation, pre-existing urinary tract infection, urological surgery, patients on anitbiotics
Intervention	Sterile urethral catheterisation	Other forms of catheterisation
Comparison	Non-sterile urethral catheterisation	Other forms of catheterisation
Outcome	Catheter associated urinary tract infection (CAUTI) confirmed by significant bacteriuria or clinical symptoms or urethral colony counts	Any other outcomes
Study design	Comparative studies: randomised controlled studies, non-randomised experimental studies and observational studies with control group	Studies without control groups

Step 5: The search strategy

Introduction

The search strategy ensures that the literature searching is as wide and thorough as is possible; thus all or most of the relevant evidence that exists and that can address the research question is identified and analysed. A comprehensive search by reducing both uncertainty and bias ensures precision and validity of the review (Khan et al 2003, pg 21–22). This step identifies the literature sources that were searched and the process of generating a search term combination for electronic database searches.

The literature sources

Both electronic and manual searches will be performed to find all the relevant studies. The grey literature, which according to Polit and Beck (2006, pg 480), consists of unpublished reports, dissertations, non-referenced publications and any other studies with similar limited distribution, were also searched for along with any ongoing research.

The electronic searches

The electronic databases shown in Table 3.2 will be searched using the search strategy list shown in Figure 3.1 (on page 51); a full explanation of the way this list was generated is in the next section of this chapter. All searches will be saved online for future reference and printed copies will be included. The hits obtained and the potentially relevant studies and their abstracts that will be found will be recorded and documented.

Table 3.2 List of electronic databases

Database	Description	Dates covered
(OVID Host)		
Journals @ Ovid Full text	OVIDONLINE	Up to Sept 02, 2008
Ovid MEDLINE(R)		1950 to August 2008
Ovid MEDLINE(R)	In-process & other non-indexed citations and Ovid MEDLINE(R)	1950 to Present
CINAHL	CINAHL – Cumulative Index to Nursing & Allied Health Literature	1982 to August 2008
AMED	Allied and Complementary Medicine	1985 to August 2008
EMBASE		1988 to Week 35 2008
EBM Reviews	All EBM Reviews – Cochrane DSR, ACP Journal Club, DARE, CCTR, CMR, HTA, and NHSEED	1991 to August 2008
BNI	British Nursing Index and Archive	1985 to August 2008

Hand searches

Manual searches will be performed by:

* scanning the reference lists of all related studies
* searching for grey literature by searching the Internet; in particular the following gateways and search engines: http://www.webarchive.org.uk/wayback/archive/20140614081921/http://www.jisc.ac.uk/whatwedo/programmes/reppres/irs.aspx (Intute Repository Search (IRS) project); https://www.shef.ac.uk/scharr (School of Health and Related Research); http://www.google.com/scholar
* searching the following search engines/databases for conference proceedings and papers, dissertations and theses, and expertise: https://portal.nihr.ac.uk; http://www.cos.com/; http://www.bl.uk
* searching for any possible ongoing research on the following databases: www.york.ac.uk/inst/crd/htadbase.htm; http://controlled-trials.com.

The search term strategy list

The list of search terms and combinations shown in Figure 3.1 will be used to search the electronic databases. It is based on the research question and its PICO components. The sensitivity of the search, which according to Khan et al (2003, pg 24) is the proportion of relevant studies, is higher when synonyms to the component terms are included in the list. It is also increased by including abbreviations and spelling variants of the terms. Khan et al (2003, pg 24) emphasise that sensitivity is a reflection of the comprehensiveness of the search. On the other hand the precision of the search, defined by Khan et al (2003, pg 27) as the number of relevant studies identified expressed as a percentage of all studies identified (relevant and not), is increased by combinations of the terms using Boolean operators and by applying limits. In order to make the search more specific, at the end of the literature search the following limits were applied: English language, human, humans and research.

Generation of the search term and combination list

The generation of the search terms and combination of lists will involve seven stages to arrive at the final search strategy list.

Stage 1: research question. The structured question will be broken down into the component parts as specified by the PICO framework: in *Patients requiring urinary catheterisation* (**P**), is *sterile catheter insertion* (**I**) more effective than *non-sterile insertion* (**C**) at reducing the incidence of *catheter associated urinary tract infections (CAUTIs)* (**O**)?

Stage 2: keywords and phrases. Using the PICO groups, keywords and phrases were identified, which are displayed in Table 3.3.

Table 3.3 Keywords and phrases

Population	Intervention	Comparison	Outcome
Patients requiring urinary catheterisation	Sterile catheter insertion	Non-sterile catheter	Catheter associated infection

Stage 3: identification of synonyms. The synonyms of the search terms that were identified can be seen in Table 3.4.

Stage 4: combining of keywords and phrases. At this step the type of study design/s was included and using Boolean operators (OR, AND, NOT) the combinations of terms will be obtained; these are presented in Table 3.5.

Stage 5: identifying abbreviations and different spelling. Possible abbreviations or spelling variants (Americanisms) of the terms in Stage 4 will be considered

⫧ **Table 3.4** Synonyms of keywords and phrases

Population	Intervention	Comparison	Outcome
Urinary catheterisation	Sterile	Non-sterile	Urinary tract infection
Urethral catheterisation	Aseptic	Clean	Bladder infection
Bladder catheterisation	Periurethral cleansing	Water	Infection
Catheterisation	Meatal cleansing	Saline	Bacteriuria
Catheter insertion	Chlorhexidine	Gloves	Asymptomatic bacteriuria
	Cetrimide		Significant bacteriuria
	Savlon		Urine dipslide
	Povidone-iodine		Dipslide
	Antiseptic solution		Urine culture
	Antiseptic		Urine sample
	Gloves		
	Gel		
	Lubricating gel		
	Antiseptic gel		
	Hand washing		
	Hand hygiene		

and the changes, displayed in Table 3.6, were obtained using truncation ($) and wild cards (?); these changes increase the sensitivity of the search.

Stage 6: constructing a search strategy table. In Table 3.7 all of the terms were numbered, starting with the first term in the first column on the left. A number was skipped on progressing from one column to the next; these numbers were then allocated to the combinations as seen in Figure 3.1.

Stage 7: translating into a search terms and combinations list. The resulting search term list can be seen in Figure 3.1. Where a search was carried out for a combination of terms, the Boolean search functions 'OR' and 'AND' are used (for example see item 6 in Figure 3.1 where OR has been used). The "?" is used as a wild card symbol. It replaces a single letter in a search word to find alternative spellings and plurals (for example orthop?dic will find both orthopaedic and orthopedic) useful to find different American spelling.

Table 3.5 Combinations of keywords and phrases

Population Boolean Operators		Intervention AND	Comparison AND	Outcome AND	Study designs AND
OR	Urinary catheterisation	Sterile	Non-sterile	Urinary tract infection	Comparative
OR	Urethral catheterisation	Aseptic	Clean	Bladder infection	Randomised
OR	Bladder catheterisation	Periurethral cleansing	Water	Infection	Controlled
OR	Catheterisation	Meatal cleansing	Saline	Bacteriuria	Quasi-randomised
OR	Catheter insertion	Chlorhexidine	Gloves	Asymptomatic bacteriuria	Observational
OR		Cetrimide		Significant bacteriuria	Study
OR		Savlon		Urine dipslide	Trial
OR		Povidone-iodine		Dipslide	Quantitative
OR		Antiseptic solution		Urine culture	RCT
OR		Antiseptic		Urine sample	
OR		Gloves			
OR		Gel			
OR		Lubricating gel			
OR		Antiseptic gel			
OR		Hand washing			
OR		Hand hygiene			

Table 3.6 Abbreviations and different spellings

Population Boolean Operators		Intervention AND	Comparison AND	Outcome AND	Study designs AND
OR	Urinary catheteri?ation	Sterile	Non-sterile	Urinary tract infection	Comparative
OR	Urethral catheteri?ation	Aseptic	Clean	Bladder infection	Randomi?$
OR	Bladder catheteri?ation	Periurethral clean?ing	Water	Infection$	Control?ed
OR	Catheteri?$	Meatal clean?ing	Saline	Bacter?uria	Quasi-randomi?ed
OR	Catheter insertion	Chlorhexidine	Glove$	Asymptomatic bacter?uria	Observational
OR		Cetrimide		Significant bacter?uria	Stud$
OR		Savlon		Urine dipslide	Trial$
OR		Povidoneiodine		Dipslide	Quantitative
OR		Antiseptic solution$		Urine culture$	RCT
OR		Antiseptic$		Urine sample$	
OR		Glove$		CAUTI	
OR		Gel		UTI	
OR		Lubricating gel			
OR		Antiseptic gel			
OR		Hand washing			
OR		Hand hygiene			

F **Table 3.7** Search strategy table

Population Boolean Operators	Intervention AND	Comparison AND	Outcome AND	Study designs AND
OR 1.Urinary catheteri?ation	7. Sterile	24. Non-sterile	30. Urinary tract infection	43. Comparative
OR 2. Urethral catheteri?ation	8. Aseptic	25. Clean	31. Bladder infection	44. Randomi?$
OR 3. Bladder catheteri?ation	9. Periurethral clean?ing	26. Water	32. Infection$	45. Control?ed
OR 4. Catheteri?$	10. Meatal clean?ing	27. Saline	33. Bacter?uria	46. Quasi-randomi?ed
OR 5. Catheter insertion	11. Chlorhexidine	28. Glove$	34. Asymptomatic bacter?uria	47.Observational
OR	12. Cetrimide		35. Significant bacter?uria	48. Stud$
OR	13. Savlon		36. Urine dipslide	49. Trial$
OR	14. Povidone-iodine		37. Dipslide	50. Quantitative
OR	15. Antiseptic solution$		38. Urine culture$	51. RCT
OR	16. Antiseptic$		39. Urine sample$	
OR	17. Glove$		40. CAUTI	
OR	18. Gel		41. UTI	
OR	19. Lubricating gel			
OR	20. Antiseptic gel			
OR	21. Hand washing			
OR	22. Hand hygiene			

The search term strategy list

1. Urinary catheteri?ation	23. 7 OR 8 OR 9 OR 10	39. Urine sample$
2. Urethral catheteri?ation	OR 11 OR 12 OR 13	40. CAUTI
3. Bladder catheteri?ation	OR 14 OR 15 OR 16	41. UTI
4. Catheteri?$	OR 17 OR 18 OR 19	42. 30 OR 31 OR 32
5. Catheter insertion	OR 20 OR 21 OR 22	OR 33 OR 34 OR 35
6. 1 OR 2 OR 3 OR 4 OR 5	24. Non-sterile	OR 36 OR 37
7. Sterile	25. Clean	OR 38 OR 39 OR 40
8. Aseptic	26. Water	OR 41
9. Periurethral clean?ing	27. Saline	43. Comparative
10. Meatal clean?ing	28. Glove$	44. Randomi?$
11. Chlorhexidine	29. 24 OR 25 OR 26 OR	45. Control?ed
12. Cetrimide	27 OR 28	46. Quasi-randomi?ed
13. Savlon	30. Urinary tract infection	47. Observational
14. Povidone-iodine	31. Bladder infection	48. Stud$
15. Antiseptic solution$	32. Infection$	49. Trial$
16. Antiseptic$	33. Bacter?uria	50. Quantitative
17. Glove$	34. Asymptomatic	51. RCT
18. Gel	bacter?uria	52. 43 OR 44 OR 45 OR
19. Lubricating gel	35. Significant bacter?uria	46 OR 47 OR 48 OR
20. Antiseptic gel	36. Urine dipslide	49 OR 50 OR 51
21. Hand washing	37. Dipslide	53. 6 AND 23 AND 29
22. Hand hygiene	38. Urine culture$	AND 42 AND 52

 Figure 3.1 The search term strategy list.

Step 6: Selecting, appraising and extracting data from your primary research papers

Introduction

This section of the report will deal with the methods of the three phases of the review: the study selection process, the assessment of the methodological qualities of the selected studies and the data extraction process. All three phases of this review will be carried out solely by the author because of restrictions of time and work constraints. Ideally two reviewers working independently should be involved in order to reduce selection bias (Torgerson 2003, pg 40). Khan et al (2003, pg 32) explain that the method of resolving any disagreements or undecided conclusions would need to be identified and would normally be clearly stated early in the protocol stage. Furthermore, agreement or consensus in most instances is reached through discussion, however, arbitration by a third person might be required if no agreed conclusion is reached.

Selection of studies

This consisted of two steps or stages. In the first step, the decision to include or exclude studies resulting from the search will be on the title and abstract only. In order to facilitate the process a standardised form will be used. This form was generated after considering the list of inclusion and exclusion criteria shown in Table 3.1 and therefore follows the PICO framework. Khan et al (2003, pg 32) highlight the probability that decisions concerning inclusion/exclusion of studies can be highly subjective and therefore lead to disagreements when more than one reviewer is involved. Therefore, the use of standardised forms serves the secondary purpose of improving inter- and intra-rater reliability by ensuring that all reviewers' assessments follow a standardised systematic approach.

In the second step, a final decision on inclusion or exclusion of the studies identified in the first stage will be made, based on reading the full text; once again a standardised form was used. The standardised forms used in the first and second selections had a similar basic layout as shown in Table 3.8 and 3.9. They consist of a list of questions that seek to identify those studies that meet the selection criteria. If all questions were answered in the affirmative, the study was included for assessment in the following phase but if all questions were answered in the negative such studies were obviously excluded. Any studies that ended up

Table 3.8 Standardized form for first selection of studies (based on title and abstracts)

Details of Study 1:

TITLE:

Authors:

Source:

Reviewer's name: Fay
Date:

	Criteria	Yes/no/undecided
Participants	Patients undergoing catheterisation?	
	Type of catheterisation: urethral, indwelling or intermittent?	
	Catheterisation performed by healthcarer?	
	Setting: hospital or nursing home?	
Intervention	Sterile/aseptic catheter insertion, non-sterile/clean catheter insertion?	
Outcome	Incidence of CAUTI or bacteriuria	
Type of study	Quantitative, comparative?	
Action (with rationale)	Include (read full article) or exclude?	

F **Table 3.9** Standardized form for second selection of studies (based on full text)

Details of Study 1:

TITLE:

Authors:

Source:

Reviewer's name: Fay
Date:

	Criteria	Yes/no
Participants	Patients undergoing catheterisation?	
	Type of catheterisation: urethral, indwelling or intermittent?	
	Catheterisation performed by healthcarer?	
	Setting: hospital or nursing home?	
Intervention	Sterile/aseptic catheter insertion, non-sterile/clean catheter insertion?	
Outcome	Incidence of CAUTI or bacteriuria	
Type of study	Quantitative, comparative?	
Action (with rationale)	Include (for full methodological analysis) or exclude?	

with an undecided conclusion in the first stage required further consideration by reading the full text before arriving at a final decision.

Assessment of methodological quality of included studies

The main objective of this assessment will be to establish the external and internal validity and reliability of the selected studies. According to Khan et al (2003, pg 126) external validity, also known as generalisability, is the extent to which the effects observed in the study can be expected to apply in routine clinical practice, whereas internal validity refers to the degree to which the results of a study are likely to approximate the truth for the participants in the study (Khan et al, 2003, pg 132). The selected studies will be quantitative, comparative studies (that have a control group). The assessment tool or checklist that will be used to analyse these studies is based on the critical review form designed by Law et al (1998) at the McMaster University that was originally intended for analysis of quantitative research studies related to occupational therapy. The adapted version of this form was chosen because it can be applied in analysis of all types of quantitative study designs and has a set of very detailed guidelines that makes it easier to use and increases its inter- and intra-rater reliability. The first page of a completed appraisal form for one of the included studies is shown in Figure 3.2.

Critical Review Form - Quantitative Studies
Law, M., Stewart, D., Pollock, N., Letts, L., Bosch, J., & Westmorland, M.

McMaster University
Adapted Word Version Used with Permission

The EB Group would like to thank Dr. Craig Scanlan, University of Medicine and Dentistry of NJ, for providing this Word version of the quantitative review form.

Instructions: Use tab or arrow keys to move between fields, mouse or spacebar to check/uncheck boxes.

CITATION	Provide the full citation for this article in APA format: Carapeti, E.A., Andrews, S.M. and Bentley, P.G. (1994) **Randomized study of sterile versus non-sterile urethral catheterisation.** *Ann R Col/ Surg Eng:* 76, pg 59–60.
STUDY PURPOSE Was the purpose stated clearly? ☒ Yes ☐ No	**Outline the purpose of the study. How does the study apply to your research question?** The purpose of this study was to assess the rate of UTI after short-term preoperative urethral catheterisation employing two different insertion techniques – sterile and non-sterile – and to compare costs. Since this paper looks at catheter insertion techniques its results can answer the question to my review.
LITERATURE Was relevant background literature reviewed? ☒ Yes ☐ No	**Describe the justification of the need for this study:** Very brief background; however it clearly justifies the need of the study by the statement of 'urethral catheterisation remains the most common cause of nosocomial infection in medical practice'. Statistically UTI account for 40% of all nosocomial infection all associated with indwelling catheterisation. It is clearly indicated that there are no studies investigating the effect of insertion technique priorto this Study.
DESIGN ☒ Randomized (RCT) ☐ cohort ☐ single case design ☐ before and after ☐ case-control ☐ cross-sectional ☐ case study	**Describe the study design. Was the design appropriate for the study question? (e.g., for knowledge level about this issue, outcomes, ethical issues, etc.):** The study design is a prospective Randomized Controlled design. This included all patients undergoing surgery and who needed to be catheterized: then patients were randomly allocated to one of the groups by a throw of a coin and then catheterized according to the instructions and methods used and according to the group these patients were allocated to. No indication of reason for catheterisation. **Specify any biases that may have been operating and the direction of their influence on the results:** Results could have been influenced by the type of catheter and the type of catheter coating used. The type of catheters used in this study is not stated.
SAMPLE N =156 Was the sample described in detail? ☒ Yes ☐ No	**Sampling (who;characteristics; how many; how was sampling done?)** **If more than one group, was there similarity between the groups?** 156 patients were included in the study, 84 females and 72 males with age range of 22 to 91 years (mean 66.8 years). The slerile technique group consisted of 74 patients with mean age of 67.5 years while the non-sterile technique group consisted of 82 patients with mean age years of 65.3 years. The authors state that there was no significant difference between groups; although the patients comparised a heterogeneous group, the two randomized

F **Figure 3.2** Completed McMaster University appraisal form (first page).

Data extraction

The data from the studies will be extracted and evaluated in an attempt to answer the review question; these data will be extracted by using a standardised data extraction form that was produced by using the PICO framework. In this form details, facts and figures regarding study characteristics, outcome and process measures were grouped under the headings Population, Intervention and Outcomes. A copy of the data extraction form can be seen in Figure 3.3.

DATA Extraction Form

Details of Study 1:

TITLE: Randomised study of sterile versus non-sterile urethral catheterisation.
        (Authors: Carapeti EA. Andrews SM. Bentley PG.)
SOURCE: *Annals of the Royal College of Surgeons of England. 78(1):59-60, 1994 Jan.*

Reviewer's Name: Fiona Bezzina   **Date:** 6 Sept 2008

Purpose of the study: to assess the rate of UTI after short-term perioperative catheterisation using sterile versus non-sterile insertion techniques and compare the costs.

Study Design: Randomised controlled trial

POPULATION:

Sample size: 156 participants (Experimental: 82, Control: 74)

Criteria of diagnosis (CAUTI or Bacteriuria): UTI defined as Bacteriuria $> 10^5$ with or without clinical symptoms

Any Secondary diagnosis: all patients underwent surgery of some form

Inclusion / Exclusion Criteria:
        Inclusion: All surgical patients.
        Exclusion: Patients with indwelling catheters, known pre-existing UTI, those undergoing lower urinary tract surgery

Type of Catheterisation: urethral, short term, perioperative

Reason for catheterisation: Not Clear

Setting: Hospital surgical theatres

INTERVENTION:

Experimental Intervention/s: Hand washing, non-sterile gloves, tap water meatal washing, KY jelly, Catheter held in plastic sheath.
Duration of Intervention/s:
Adverse Effects: None reported

Control Treatment/s: Hand scrubbing, Gown, Sterile gloves, Sterile pack, No-touch technique, Savlon meatal cleansing, Sterile drapes, Sterile lignocaine gel, insertion with forceps
Drop-outs: None Reported

Study 1: Carapeti et al (1994):   DATA Extraction Form (Continued)

<u>**OUTCOMES:**</u>

CAUTI:

Number of UTI's (in Experimental and Control groups):

  Bacteriuria (Urine sample]: not specified
  Symptomatic UTI: not specified
  Combined Results: Experimental: 9
                    Control: 7
Types of Infecting Organisms: none specified

Time of Urine Sample / UTI (from Catheter insertion):
          First sample collected at insertion.
          Second sample 3 days post-insertion.

CAUTI Incidence Rate (as percentage) in:
          Intervention Group: 11%
          Control Group: 9.5%
          Statistical significance: *P>0.1*

UTI Rate according to Gender: UTI was present in 11.9% of females and in 8.3% of males
                    (*P>0.1*)

 Figure 3.3 Data extraction form.

📝 *Step 7: Plans for synthesizing the data (Chapter10)*

Box 3.2   Checklist you can use to assess whether you have included all sections of your protocol

---

Title and question

Is the title a true representation of the content?

Are all components of the question included within the title?

Has an appropriate question relevant to the area of expertise been developed?

Abstract

Is there a clear summary of the research including the background, objectives (and rationale), procedures, results, conclusions and implications to the field? Abstract no more than 300–400 words.

Background

- Is the background to the area well written and would it be considered capable of promoting interest?
- Has the importance of the problem been highlighted and appropriate references used?
- Is there an explanation of how the review extends the existing literature? Or if it is a duplication of another review is it clear how the student's review is different?
- Relevance of the study to the field or gap in knowledge. That is, the student needs to show that no review exactly like theirs has been carried out.
- Does it demonstrate some knowledge of the specialist area of practice and question orthodox practice using balanced, logical and supported argument?
- Is independence of thought and open-mindedness demonstrated?

Objectives and aims

- Statement of the study's objective/s (or if relevant hypotheses).
- Are the objectives (or research question) based on the background?
- Is it clear how these objectives will be measured?
- Are they relevant to the clinical area under investigation?

Criteria for considering studies in review

This should follow from the research question:

- Have details of the types of participants to be included in the review been described?
- Have details been given of the types of intervention (exposure or test to be evaluated)?
- Have details been given of the types of comparative groups (or gold standard reference test) to be included in review?
- Have details been given of the types of study (designs) to be included in review?
- Have details been given of the types of outcome measures to be included in review?

Search strategy

- Are the PICO or PEO Outcome) components of the research question identified?
- Is it clear how the student derived all the synonyms from the research question and used Boolean operators appropriately to enable the formulation of the search strategy?
- Are all databases to be searched described and the dates provided?
- Are all possible sources of literature to be searched? For example: electronic databases, MEDLINE, EMBASE, PsychLIT, CINAHL, etc?
- Are specialist trial registers checked? Cochrane?

(Continued)

Box 3.2   Continued

- Is hand searching to be undertaken?
- Are reference lists to be checked?
- Is grey literature to be checked? For example, PhDs and BScs in libraries, conference proceedings or abstracts?
- Is the description of the search strategy detailed enough to the extent that someone else could duplicate it and get the same results?
- Overall is the search efficient and used appropriately?

Methods

Have details of all three parts of the methods section been described?

Part 1: the process of selecting papers for inclusion in the review. This process consists of two steps: the initial paper selection followed by the second more thorough selection of papers.

First selection of papers:

- Is the first selection of papers (for inclusion in review) based on titles and abstracts only?
- Is the student to conduct it alone or are two students to perform it independently? If alone have they stated how this would impact on the validity of the results?
- Are the procedures to be used going to be tested on a sample of articles (somewhat like a pilot study)?
- Was a standardized form made for this procedure? Is it appropriate and adequate to answer the research question?
- Was a clear description provided of the criteria the students were looking for at this stage?
- Is it clear how disagreements will be resolved (if more than one student)?

Second (more thorough) selection of papers: the criteria for this section are the same as above except that the selection of papers is based on reading the whole paper.

Part 2: the procedure for the assessment of methodological quality

- Is the appropriate checklist used to assess the methodological quality of each paper included in the assignment? For example, if student used RCTs, controlled clinical trials (CCTs) and qualitative papers, then three checklists need to be included and described in this section.
- Are the checklists to be used well cited and referenced?
- Is it clear how many people are to assess the studies and how this is to be carried out?
- Are assessments to be done independently?
- Is a description given of how the papers are to be marked? For example, using a numerical scale or other such as very poor, poor, adequate, good, very good.

(Continued)

The data extraction strategy

- Is the appropriate data to be extracted to enable the research question to be answered?
- Is the standardized form used to extract data appropriate to collect all the data necessary to answer the research question?
- Is the data extraction form to be piloted in any way before it is used in the study?
- Is data to be extracted by one or more than one student? Has student discussed the implications?
- How are disagreements to be resolved if more than one student?

References

- Was the Harvard format used?
- Do citations and references match?
- Accurately presented?
- Wide range and scope of papers?

Presentation

- Was the correct layout used for title page, contents, page numbers, etc. (see these guidelines)?
- Text free from errors and spelling mistakes?
- Appropriate use of vocabulary and grammar?
- Appropriate use of the appendices?
- Logical and clear presentation of appendices?
- Clear and aesthetic style and presentation of the report as a whole?

🔑 Key points

When writing your own protocol the following key points should be considered.

- Before your start writing the full review it is very important to search a number of websites where you can check if another systematic literature review of your exact review question has already been done. It would be very disappointing to have done your review and then find someone else has just conducted the same review a few months ago.

- Before your start writing the full review it is very important to write a protocol or plan for your review.

- This is important because it enables you to identify your question, inclusion and exclusion criteria, objective etc . . . offering a structured and systematic approach to undertaking your review. The aim is to identify any potential issues before you commence your review.

- Start with the background discussion.

- Clearly state your objects (primary and secondary if needed).

- Describe the steps you plan to take to conduct your review, that is, how will you search for, select, appraise and extract data from your research papers to enable you to answer your review question.
- Be sure to include a copy of the forms to (1) select your papers, (2) assess the methodology of your included papers and (3) extract data from your papers within your protocol.
- Finally be sure to finish by describing briefly how you plan to synthesize the data you extract.

Summary

This chapter has discussed the importance of writing a protocol for your review and described the steps you need to take when planning your review. We have also included a number of websites where you can check if another systematic literature review of your exact review question has already been done. A brief overview of all the steps/sections to include within your protocol was described and an example of a real student's protocol was provided.

Question and Answer (Q&A)

(Q) What are the important messages to learn from Fay's protocol?

(A) Following a recognized framework for developing the protocol will serve to enhance the quality and outcome of your systematic review.

- It makes the work for conducting the review much easier.
- It will help you make sure that you don't change the way you conduct the full review once you have started it.
- It reduces bias.
- It enables replication.

4

Writing the background to your review

Overview

- Background to your protocol
- Providing an operational definition of the clinical problem
- Highlighting the importance of the review question and grabbing the attention of the reader
- Clarifying the gap in systematic reviews in the clinical area
- Using different tools and methods to help you start writing up your background section
- The importance of managing and planning your time

Background to your protocol

The role of the background in your protocol (and later in the review) is to describe the setting and context of the area of research, the importance of the topic and the reasons why it has been chosen (Higgins and Green 2011). There may be a number of reasons for the choice of topic, for example reporting a review to evaluate the effectiveness of a particular treatment or replicating an important review in a particular area of practice carried out in another country or a number of years previously.

A well-written background should be clear about the direction of the study. In the background, it is important to explain what reviews have already been conducted in this area, if any, discuss their strengths and limitations, and describe how the proposed review will fill a gap in the literature, providing new information that could advance practice (Cochrane Collaboration 2009).

It is important not to be too anecdotal in recounting the reasons for conducting the review. Back up your reasons with facts and figures and references where possible. For an intervention study, the background could include some or all of the following, depending on the specific topic of your review.

1 Provide an operational definition of the clinical problem.
2 Cite research papers or government documents with statistical figures to highlight the importance of the study.
4 Describe the signs and symptoms (or consequences) of the disease, illness, problem or issue.
4 Provide details of the patients' age, gender and other pertinent details.
5 Describe the course of the disease or pathophysiology.

6 If the review is related to the effectiveness of any type of intervention, there needs to be a discussion about how the disease or issue is usually managed in practice.

7 Describe the general outcome measures.

8 Once the problem has been discussed, including incidence, effect on patients' lives and management, a gap in systematic reviews in the evidence or literature needs to be identified. References should be used to support how the proposed review is different.

Remember that you are trying to show that there is a gap in systematic literature reviews and not in primary research papers or narrative reviews. Some of the key issues will now be discussed individually and in more depth.

Providing an operational definition of the clinical problem

When starting the background section it is usual to provide an 'operational definition' of the clinical problem you are addressing in your review. An operational definition is a clear, concise, detailed definition of a measure described within a particular context; here you will be stating what the problem is and what it is not. Once you have provided an operational definition and if your issue relates to a clinical problem, it is usually appropriate to describe the following: the causes of the condition, the age of your specific population group, the specific diagnosis, the signs and symptoms of the illness or problem, and the natural history or course of the disease or pathophysiology.

ℂ In Cheryl's example on bracing for adolescents with scoliosis, in her background section, Cheryl needs to provide an operational definition of the term 'adolescent idiopathic scoliosis (AIS)' to clarify the nature of the clinical problem. Cheryl could write something like the paragraph below. After every statement, it is important to include a reference to demonstrate that this piece of information has been obtained from a reliable source.

> Adolescent Idiopathic Scoliosis is a deformity of the spine and rib cage which generally occurs in children and adolescents between the ages of 10–16 years old (Parent 2005). The causes of AIS are not known though many theories have been put forward over the years; these include possible genetic, muscular or neurological causes among others (Scoliosis Research Society (SRS) 2006).

Highlighting the importance of the review question and grabbing the attention of the reader

There are a number of ways to clarify the importance of the research or clinical problem, including the use of statistics, key government papers and previous important research work in the area. The use of statistics highlights the importance of the problem within the general population. The statement 'Low back pain occurs in 80 per cent of the population at some time in their lives' makes it clear that low back pain is an important clinical problem. Citing key government documents within your background is a good strategy as it demonstrates the importance that government bodies allocate to this specific area of health. For example, Cheryl could write something like this:

> The incidence of AIS varies between different countries from 0.9 to 12 per cent (Parent 2005). AIS occurs much more frequently in girls and for curves of over 40 degrees and the occurrence of adolescent idiopathic scoliosis in girls as compared with boys is approximately 8:2 or four times greater (Bates 2010).

In the example above, the statement that AIS can occur in up to 12 per cent of children and mainly in girls is highlighting that this is an important problem that needs to be reviewed. Once the importance of the topic has been clarified, the signs and symptoms of the clinical condition could be discussed. In Cheryl's example, she could say something like the following.

> The deformity results in a spinal curvature together with a rib hump and shoulder, waist and pelvic asymmetries (Lonstein 2006). This deformity has a significant impact on these young children and adolescents. These include a decreased quality of life as well as many psychological problems such as low self-esteem and self-image (Maclean 1989; Freidel 2002).

Once Cheryl has discussed the clinical problem together with the resultant signs and symptoms of the condition, it is appropriate for her to discuss the current management for patients with AIS.

> Patients with AIS are generally treated to prevent the curvature and rib hump getting any worse. The treatment type depends on the severity of the curvature and rib hump. For small curves (10–40 degrees) either annual monitoring and observation or scoliosis-specific exercises are usually recommended. Curves between 40 and 50 degrees are usually braced or observed and curves over 50 degrees are usually recommended for surgery.

Practical Tip

Detailing the background and context to your clinical problem with the backing of robust evidence is a good way of obtaining the backing from nurse leaders, managers and commissioners to support the review.

Clarifying the gap in systematic reviews in the clinical area

Describing and briefly critiquing previous reviews that have been conducted in your specific review area is important. You need to show that your systematic review has not been conducted before and that yours is the most up-to-date and best quality review. If narrative reviews have been conducted in your specific area, it is worth mentioning them but explaining that as they are narrative reviews the results may be biased. If there are previous systematic reviews you would like to include, you should provide a brief description and explain what was reviewed and when, and then very clearly point out how your review is different from these. In other words you are attempting to clarify the gap in systematic reviews in the literature.

This is important because your aim is to prove that your systematic review is actually needed. If an identical review was carried out over a year ago and no primary papers in this area have been published since then, it is clear that a systematic review would not be needed. In order to show the gap in systematic reviews in your specific area, you now need to describe what other reviews have been conducted, whether they were narrative or systematic reviews, how long ago they were conducted, and to what extent your review is similar or different. Returning to Cheryl's example.

> To date, reviews in this area have been mostly narrative reviews that have not included the evaluation of the methodological quality of the included studies and have not included all relevant primary papers. For example, the narrative review by Chan (2004) did not include all primary papers in the area and the narrative review by Ottenburger (2007) did not evaluate the methodological quality of the included primary papers. One systematic review was found but this related to the effect of braces on adults and not adolescents with idiopathic scoliosis. A 'gold standard' systematic review is needed to make sure that the 'sacrifices that children are making when wearing a brace are indeed worthwhile' (Negrini 2010: 4).

All the above excerpts are based on a Cochrane Review on *Braces for Idiopathic Scoliosis in Adolescents*, which I undertook together with a team of international researchers (Negrini et al. 2010). Should you wish to read the whole background of this review you can find it at: http://onlinelibrary.wiley.com/doi/10.1002/14651858.CD006850.pub2/pdf

Cheryl's examples are based on this review, but I would like to clarify that I have added or changed some sentences in order to illustrate a point or make an argument. In our case no systematic reviews that specifically addressed the effectiveness of braces on adolescents with idiopathic scoliosis had as yet been undertaken.

Using different tools and methods to help you start writing up your background section

There are a number of different tools that you can use to help you write up the background section of your review. In the case study, Cheryl is aware that if she begins writing too soon she will be forced to stop and go back to the initial steps. Cheryl has searched widely and has read a number of review papers, government documents and research papers in the general area of AIS. She has also been trying to identify what is known and what is not known about her topic. She will begin to write her protocol only when she is confident that she can answer 'Yes' to the six questions listed in Box 4.1.

Practice session 4.1

Complete Box 4.1 for your own review.

Box 4.1   Template to complete for your background section

Have you searched and read broadly in the area of your specific review question?	YES ☐	NO ☐
Have you made sure that a number of primary research papers have been conducted relating to your specific area of interest?	YES ☐	NO ☐
Have you spent time thinking critically about your specific review topic?	YES ☐	NO ☐
Have you spent time discussing your review topic with your colleagues or supervisor with a knowledge of this area?	YES ☐	NO ☐
Have you found out how people in other disciplines think about your research topic?	YES ☐	NO ☐
Do you feel ready to begin writing your research protocol?	YES ☐	NO ☐

Before you start writing the background to your review, it is important that you have read around the area and spoken to your colleagues or supervisors about it. Creating a mind map, making lists and brainstorming are useful tools to get you started. Try answering the questions in Box 4.1 before you start to check that you are ready to start writing your background. Many clinicians and students undertaking a systematic literature review in nursing for the first time are unsure about how and where to start. A good way round this is to try to draw a mind map. Mind mapping is a process of representing 'concepts' or knowledge structures used in learning in a two-dimensional graphic arrangement and includes the labelling and linking of concepts to form associations or hierarchies. The centre represents the hub or central theme.

By presenting ideas in a radial, graphical, non-linear manner, mind maps encourage a brainstorming approach to planning and organizational tasks (Rooda 1994). Brainstorming is a creativity technique in which a group of people try to find a solution for a specific problem by gathering a list of ideas spontaneously contributed by its members. Although Cheryl could do this activity on her own, she decides to get together with a group of her colleagues (as they may have ideas and thoughts about the topic that she may not have thought about) to begin drawing a mind map on the topic of braces for scoliosis (Figure 4.1).

Practical Tip

There are numerous software packages available that can help you to develop your own ideas and mind maps. In some instances these can be obtained free online, and can help support you in presenting your ideas/findings in a visual way. Before you begin mind mapping ensure you familiarize yourself with the software, it will save you time later.

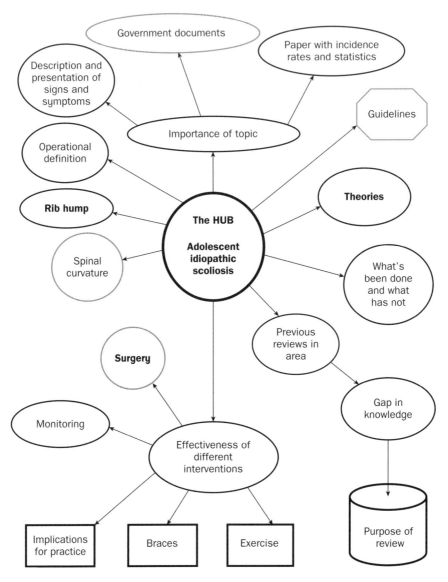

Figure 4.1 Example of a mind map that Cheryl could make on her topic of braces for scoliosis.

Practice session 4.2

Try to make a mind map for your own review topic in Box 4.2.

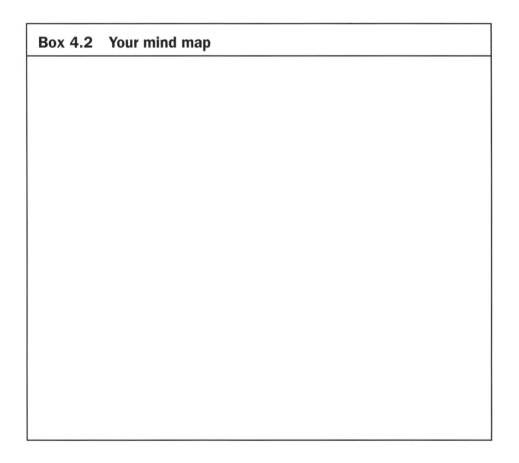

See Figure 4.2 for how Cheryl has organized her mind map.

Alternative template

If you prefer, you can use a list instead of a mind map to write the topics you would like to include in your background, listing each issue one beneath the other in the same order that you will write them in your own background. An example is detailed below.

Ⓒ

1   Definition of AIS.
2   Description and presentation.
4   Importance of topic.
4   Effect on people's lives.

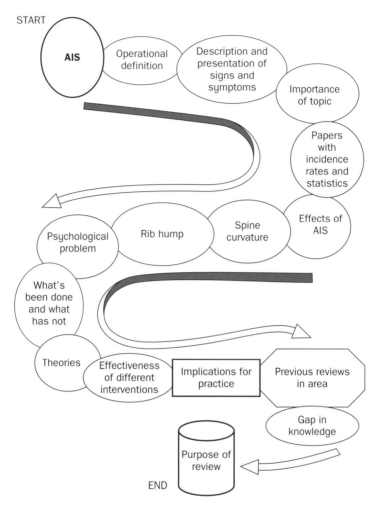

Figure 4.2 Cheryl organizes her mind map in the order she plans to write it up.

5   Previous research in area.

6   Theories.

7   Effectiveness of different interventions.

8   Gap in knowledge.

9   Purpose.

Practice session 4.3

In Box 4.3 try to organize your mind map in the order that you plan to write it out.

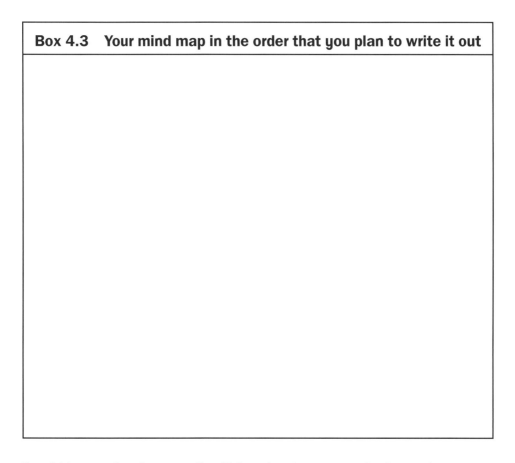

Box 4.3   Your mind map in the order that you plan to write it out

Box 4.4 is a template for you to list all the points for your own background.

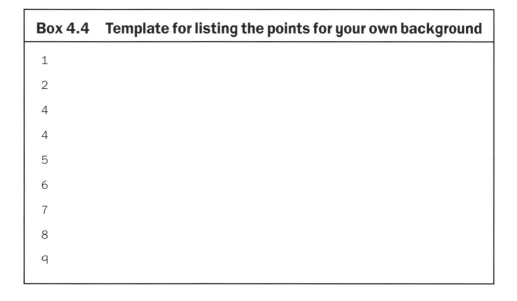

Box 4.4   Template for listing the points for your own background

1
2
4
4
5
6
7
8
9

Once Cheryl has made a list of all the concepts, she decides to add another column to her list. In this column she writes all the possible sources of information that she may require and makes sure that they are available nearby so she can refer to them as she writes. Table 4.1 shows Cheryl's new list. Box 4.5 provides a template for you to list your own themes and possible sources of information.

Ɛ **Table 4.1** Cheryl's themes and possible sources of information

	Themes	Possible sources of information and activities to do
1	Definition of AIS	Dictionary Government documents Review documents Research papers
2	Description and presentation	As above
4	Importance of topic	Papers with statistics and incidence rates Government health department documents
4	Effect on people's lives	All above, especially research papers and reviews
5	Previous research in area	Research papers and systematic reviews or other reviews that have done research in a similar or related area
6	Theories	Theoretical papers or research papers primarily
7	Effectiveness of different interventions	Research papers showing effectiveness of different intervention studies
8	Gap in knowledge	All above, highlighting what has and has not been done yet
٩	Purpose	This will address the gap above

Ƒ *Commentary on Fay's 'background' section*

To go back to what was said above on pages 61 and 62 of this chapter, these are some of the points that could be included in your background section especially if you are conducting a systematic review on an intervention. On the next page you will find a few excerpts from Fay's background section and next to each excerpt is the point (or number below) that it is addressing. We would suggest you refer to the protocol in the previous section (Chapter 3) to remind yourself of where these excerpts 'sit' within the background section. So to repeat what we said on pages 61 and 62 of this chapter, your background could include some or all of the following, depending on the specific topic of your review.

1 Provide an operational definition of the clinical problem.

2 Cite research papers or government documents with statistical figures to highlight the importance of the study.

Box 4.5   Template for listing your own themes and possible sources of information

	Themes	Possible sources of information
1	Operational definition	
2		
3		
4		
5		
6		
7		
8		
9		

3 Describe the signs and symptoms (or consequences) of the disease, illness, problem or issue.

4 Provide details of the patients' age, gender and other pertinent details.

5 Describe the course of the disease or pathophysiology.

6 If the review is related to the effectiveness of any type of intervention, there needs to be a discussion about how the disease or issue is usually managed in practice.

7 Describe the general outcome measures.

8 Once the problem has been discussed, including incidence, effect on patients' lives and management, *a gap in systematic reviews in the evidence or literature needs to be identified*. References should be used to support how the proposed review is different from other systematic reviews in the area.

Below you will find examples of actual excerpts from Fay's background section that are in italic text and the original text can be found within her proposal in the previous Chapter 3 in pages 8–10. Please note that the number icons within the box refer to the number of the point above (on page 61 and 62) that the excerpt is addressing.

Example 1

> 1 *Hospital acquired infection can be defined as an infection that is neither present, nor incubating, at the time of admission to hospital (Hospital Acquired Infection [online]).*

Commentary: Fay starts by offering a general operational definition (a definition that explains 'what something is' within the context within which you are using it; these are very important to state in order to ensure that all readers of your work understand specifically what you are talking about) of what hospital acquired infection is and later focuses this to define what CAUTI is in practice. It is a good idea to provide a definition(s) of your clinical area of concern as soon as possible in the background (point 1 above).

Example 2

> 2 *Urinary catheterisation of patients is a common nursing procedure used both in the hospital and in the community. According to Dougherty and Lister (2004, pg 444) catheter associated infections are the most common nosocomial infection, counting up to around 45% of all hospital acquired infections.*

Commentary: Fay starts her background by showing us the importance of her topic and letting the reader know that CAUTIs are very common. She also strengthens her statement by letting us know that they make up 45% of hospital acquired infections and backs this up using a reference (point 2 above).

Example 3

> 2 *Studies by Bryan and Reynolds (1984, pg 494–498) and Turck and Stamm, (1981, pg 651–654) concluded that between 75% and 80% of all healthcare associated UTIs follow the insertion of a urinary catheter and a study by Glynn et al (1997) which investigated 40 English hospitals, estimated that around 26% of all hospitalised patients have a urinary catheter inserted, whilst Parker (1999, pg 564–574) and Godfrey and Evans (2000, pg 682–690) suggest that 4% of patients in the community, at some point, will have a catheter inserted.*

Commentary: Fay goes a step further here and provides the statistics and references to show that up to 80% of healthcare UTIs follow the insertion of a urinary catheter. This statement suggests (to some degree at least) that had the catheter not been inserted or had further care or a more sterile environment been used, these infections may have been prevented. In other words Fay is further highlighting the huge importance of this issue to healthcare both in hospitals as well as in the community.

Example 4

> 3, 2 & 5 *Furthermore, complications that may arise from urinary catheterisation include structural damage to the urinary tract, bleeding, false passage, and urinary tract infections and bacteriuria (Joanna Briggs online).*

Commentary: By describing all the complications (point 3) that can arise from the insertion of a catheter Fay is again highlighting the importance of her research question within the area of healthcare (point 2). She is also describing the course of the disease or pathophysiology (point 5).

Example 5

> 2 *It is estimated that CAUTI costs the National Health Service (NHS) £1,427 per patient and because it increases the period of hospitalisation of such patients, by approximately three to six days, costs approximately increase by £124 million per year (Hart, 2008, pg 44–48; SSHAIP, 2004, [online]).*

Commentary: By providing the actual figures as to the increased costs that CAUTI can result in Fay is again highlighting the big importance of this clinical problem and suggesting that this issue needs to be looked at urgently. By detailing this information Fay may receive support from nurse leaders, managers and commissioners to do the review.

Example 6

> 1 *A catheter is a tubular device which is passed through the urethra into the bladder in order to drain urine or to instill medical treatment (Dougherty and Lister, 2004, pg 440–444; Steward, in BJN monograph, 2001, pg 42).*

Commentary: Here Fay is providing the reader with the operational definitions of what a catheter is and when it should be used. As discusssed above, an operational definition is a definition that explains 'what something is' within the context within which you are using it. These are very important to state so as to make sure that all readers of your work understand specifically what you are talking about. In other words to use very colloquial terminology, make sure that 'everyone is singing from the same hymn sheet'.

Example 7

> 6 *Catheterisation is indicated in and used to relieve obstructed flow of urine, to measure the residual amount in the bladder, to provide post-operative drainage following bladder, vaginal and prostate surgery, in monitoring hourly urine output in the critically ill patient, and in continence care (Brunner and Suddarth, 1992, pg 682; Steward, in BJN monograph, 2001, pg 42). Insertion of a urinary catheter is a common procedure in both acute and primary care settings, and careful consideration is always required over the need for, versus, the risk of this procedure.*

Commentary: Here Fay is describing when and why catheterization is used – again to clarify for the reader the situations when it is needed. You will note that she mentions that 'careful' consideration is always required over the need for, versus, the risk of this procedure as complications and infections are so common (as she mentioned above).

Example 8

> 6 & 2 *Urethral catheterisation may be performed as an indwelling or an intermittent procedure. Indwelling catheterisation consists of continuous catheter drainage which can be sub-classified into short term (1–7 days), mid term*

(7–28 days) and long term (28 days up to 4 months) (Hart, 2008, pg 44–48; Head, 2006, pg 44–46; RCN, 2008, pg 2–55). Intermittent catheterisation consists of epi-sodic introduction of a catheter into the bladder to drain urine out (Dougherty and Lister, 2004, pg 445). The catheter is passed via the urethra and removed soon after the bladder urine is drained. In recent years this technique has become noticeably popular, and can be carried out by the patient him/herself or by the nurse. This form of catheterisation is indicated for the drainage of a poorly functioning bladder (as is found in spinal cord injury patients and those with neurological disorders) and for the urinary drainage in the peri-operative period. Its main advantage is that the patient is left catheter-free in between catheterisations (Dougherty and Lister, 2004, pg 445; Robinson, 2007, pg 48–56). Intermittent catheterisation is also com-monly used to instill medications, measure residual urine, and it is also used to instill contrast material into the bladder to study the bladder and the urethra (Hart, 2008, pg 44–48). Lapides et al (2002, pg 1584–1586) and Wilson (1998, pg S10–14) advocate that this procedure should be undertaken as a sterile procedure in the hos-pital environment due to the high risk of hospital acquired infections, while in the community a clean technique should be used.

Commentary: Fay is now describing the different types of catheterization (in other words the different types of the intervention that are available and how the intervention is applied) (point 6). She is also using numerous references to support her statements and illustrating the use of (point 2) above.

Example 9

5 *CAUTI is asymptomatic in the majority of cases (Tambyah et al, 2000, pg 678–682); however, Godfrey and Evans (2000, pg 682–690) clarify that CAUTI can present with signs and symptoms such as: pyrexia, pyuria, uri-nary bypassing of the catheter, cloudy foul-smelling urine, confusion in elderly patients, haematuria and back pain.*

Commentary: Fay clearly defines what CAUTI is and the associated signs and symptoms.

Example 10

4 *These symptoms may vary with the age and sex of the patient and also with the severity and site of the infection. Pickerman (1994, pg 66–68) suggests that these signs and symptoms occur when the bacteria invade the bladder mucosa resulting in inflammation. Diagnosis is established after obtaining a urine sample for culture and sensitivity.*

Commentary: Fay makes it clear that the signs and symptoms may vary with age, gen-der and location of the infection. She also makes it clear how the diagnosis is obtained.

Example 11

> 7 *A bacterial count of 100,000 organisms (or CFU) per millilitre is considered to be significant of urinary tract infection. Bacteriuria and urinary tract infection are two terms used interchangeably in the nursing literature. Bacteriuria is the presence of bacteria in the urine; however, according to Higgins (1995, pg 44–45) bacteriuria in patients with indwelling and intermittent catheters does not always suggest a diagnosis of urinary tract infection (UTI).*

Commentary: In this paragraph Fay describes what exactly constitutes a significant bacterial infection and how this may present itself clinically. Fay also describes how this outcome is measured objectively per millilitre, that is a bacterial count of 100,000 organisms (or CFU) per millilitre.

Example 12

> 8 *Three systematic reviews were identified in the literature. The review by Jamison et al (2004) focuses mainly on the use of catheter types in management of the neurogenic bladder whereas the review by Niel-Weise and van den Broek (2005) looked at studies comparing urethral indwelling, intermittent and supra-pubic catheterisation. The review by Lockwood et al (2004, pg 271–291) treated the issue of sterility at insertion very briefly; only two relevant studies were included. Since these reviews focused mainly on other catheter related matters, their search strategy, therefore, could have resulted in studies relevant to the antiseptic issue being missed and left out. This study focused solely on this particular issue of sterility at catheter insertion and adopted a search strategy that would include as many of the studies that specifically dealt with this topic.*

Commentary: This highlights the importance of identifying a knowledge deficit (gap) within existing systematic reviews. This is imperative because it highlights the importance of your systematic review within the existing evidence base.

The importance of managing and planning your time

Conducting a systematic review is a time-consuming process and it is vital that you set aside enough time to conduct it. If you are writing a systematic review dissertation, you will have been given specific criteria to write this and you will need a significant period (2–4 months minimum) depending on how much time you can devote to conducting it and writing it up. If you are conducting a systematic review as part of your continuing professional development, you should set aside at least 3–4 months just to

Table 4.2 Example of a Gantt chart

Weeks	1	2	3	4	5	6	7	8	9
Select an area and carry out background reading	▓	▓							
Develop a question		▓	▓						
Write the background			▓	▓	▓				
Write the objectives					▓				
Write the criteria					▓				
Select your studies						▓			
Appraise your studies						▓	▓		
Extract data							▓		
Write results								▓	
Write discussion								▓	▓
Write up paper or dissertation								▓	▓

write your plan and protocol and then possibly another 6–12 months to conduct it and write it all up. We usually advise our students to make a timetable of all the activities involved and set a deadline for each activity. A Gantt chart is a useful tool to use and can help significantly in making sure you stick to your deadlines (see Table 4.2). You can use the Gantt chart in Box 4.6 for your own systematic review; you may want to change the word 'weeks' to 'months'.

Practical Tip

If you can demonstrate that your review is linked to resolving an existing clinical problem/need you may be able to use this to negotiate some time to undertake the review with your nurse leaders/managers and/or commissioners.

Box 4.6   Template Gantt chart for your own systematic review

Weeks	1	2	3	4	5	6	7	8	9
Select an area and carry out background reading									
Develop a question									
Write the background									
Write the objectives									
Write the criteria									
Select your studies									
Appraise your studies									
Extract data									
Write results									
Write discussion									
Write up paper or dissertation									

✐ Key points

- Writing a plan of what you intend to include before you start your systematic review is very important.

- A plan describes in advance the review question and your rationale for the proposed methods you will use. It also includes details of how different types of studies will be located, appraised and synthesized.

- Once you have formulated your review question, it is a good idea to undertake a quick general search (also called a scoping search) to make sure that there are no systematic literature reviews already available or in progress that have addressed your review question.

- A plan includes all of the following sections:
  - an answerable review question
  - the background to the review
  - the objectives of the review
  - the inclusion and exclusion criteria
  - the search strategy
  - the proposed methods for selecting, appraising and extracting the relevant data from your research papers to answer your review question.

- The background in the protocol (and later in the review) is to describe the setting and context of the area of research, the importance of the topic and the reasons why it has been chosen. In the background section of your protocol, you may consider including some of the following:
  - provide an operational definition of the clinical problem
  - cite research papers or government documents with statistical figures to highlight the importance of the study
  - describe the signs and symptoms of the disease
  - provide details of the patients' age, gender and other pertinent details
  - describe the course of the disease
  - if the review is related to the effectiveness of any type of intervention, there needs to be a discussion about how the disease or issue is usually managed in practice
  - describe the general outcome measures
  - a systematic review gap in the evidence or literature needs to be identified
  - references should be used to support how the proposed review is different.

- There are a number of different tools such as mind maps and lists that you can use to help you write up the background section of your review.

Summary

This chapter discussed the key factors that need to be considered when writing a plan for your systematic literature review. The different sections within the plan were briefly described and examples provided. The first stage of the plan, the background, was discussed in more detail and excerpts included to clarify this process. Different tools and methods were suggested to help you start writing up the background section of your plan.

Question and Answer (Q&A)

(Q) Why is the background section to the review so time consuming?

(A) Taking the time to research and detail the background and context to why your review is important will have a huge impact on the outcome of the final review. For example, it takes time to obtain, review, collate and synthesize policy documents, recent evidence, statistics, facts and figures.

Taking the time to develop a robust background will also help you to highlight to nurse leaders, mangers and commissioners why the review is needed and may secure financial backing and support for you to undertake it.

5

Specifying your objectives and inclusion and exclusion criteria

Overview

- Clarifying the preliminaries: problem statement, review question, aims and objectives
- Stating your aims and objectives
- Issues to consider when writing your problem statement, aims, objectives, review question and title
- Specifying the inclusion and exclusion criteria for selecting your primary research papers

Clarifying the preliminaries: problem statement, review question, aims and objectives

To avoid making mistakes when undertaking a review, it is important to be clear regarding the precise meaning and the differences between a problem statement, a review question, an aim and an objective. Depending on which papers or books you read, these terms may sometimes be used interchangeably. This occurs quite frequently with the terms 'objectives' and 'aims', which actually have slightly different meanings.

A problem statement is usually a simple statement of 'what is'. For example, 'It is not known if treatment 1 or treatment 2 is more effective for treating adult patients with chronic obstructive pulmonary disease (COPD)'. A problem statement means that you are simply *stating* a problem.

The review question usually follows from the problem and the problem statement. This involves changing the problem statement into a review question. Consider this problem statement: 'It is not known if treatment 1 or treatment 2 is more effective for treating adult patients with COPD'. To change this statement into a review question, all you need to do is rephrase the statement into a question like this: 'Is treatment 1 or treatment 2 more effective in treating adult patients with COPD?' The easiest way to do this is to use similar or even identical terminology to ensure that there is no change in meaning between the problem statement and the review question.

Once you have written the review question, how are the aims and objectives derived? In most dictionaries you will find that the terms 'aim' and 'objective' are synonyms (that is, words meaning the same thing), with both terms referring to the purpose for doing something. Within the area of research methodology, these terms tend to be used for different types of research. The term 'aim' is usually used to state the purpose of a study within qualitative research studies whereas the term 'objective' is generally used in quantitative research. You will find when you have read numerous papers that this is not always the case and in many reviews these terms are also used interchangeably.

The 'aim' of a project is to solve the problem and answer the question, and is usually a general statement (Jenkins et al. 1998), whereas the term 'objective' is more specific than the aim. The objectives usually state what the researcher is going to do. For every aim, there are usually two or more objectives. In the example above, 'Is treatment 1 or treatment 2 more effective in treating adult patients with COPD?' there are a number of activities that the researcher will need to do. See box 5.1 below.

Box 5.1   COPD example relating to the effectiveness of treatments for patients with COPD

Problem statement
It is not known if treatment 1 or treatment 2 is more effective for treating patients with COPD.

Review question
Is treatment 1 or treatment 2 more effective for treating patients with COPD?

Aim
The aim of this study is to evaluate if there is a difference between treatment 1 and treatment 2 for patients with COPD.

Objectives
- Collect data on the effectiveness of treatment 1 and treatment 2.
- Compare the effectiveness of the two treatments.
- Compare the findings of this study with other studies.
- Provide recommendations/guidelines for helping patients with COPD.

Title of review
A systematic literature review comparing the effectiveness of treatment 1 to treatment 2 for treating patients with COPD

So if we now refer back to Cheryl's scoliosis example, an aim is a more general statement while the objectives are much more specific (see Box 5.2).

Stating your aims and objectives

Once you have written a first draft of the background (detailed in Chapter 4) for your review, you will need to state the aim or aims and the objectives for your review. It is important that the aims and objectives include all the PICO (or PEO) elements in the same way as they are included for the review question.

🅒 Box 5.2   Cheryl's example relating to the effectiveness of treatments for adolescent patients with scoliosis

Problem statement

It is not known if treatment 1 or treatment 2 is more effective for treating adolescent patients with scoliosis.

Review question

Is treatment 1 or treatment 2 more effective for treating adolescent patients with scoliosis?

Aim

The aim of this study is to evaluate if there is a difference between treatment 1 and treatment 2 for adolescent patients with scoliosis.

Objectives

- Collect data on the effectiveness of treatment 1 and treatment 2.
- Compare the effectiveness of the two treatments.
- Compare the findings of this study with other studies.
- Provide guidelines for helping adolescent patients with scoliosis.

Title of review

A systematic literature review comparing the effectiveness of treatment 1 to treatment 2 for treating adolescent patients with scoliosis.

Practical Tip

Remember the aim is a general statement to outline a problem and the objective is a series of statements about how you intend to address the problem. Think in terms of what you, the researcher, are going to be doing (specifically what activities) to complete the systematic review.

🅒 Let's refer back to Cheryl's question: 'In patients with adolescent idiopathic scoliosis how effective is spinal bracing as compared with other treatments at reducing spinal curvature, rib hump and psychological problems?' Cheryl's aim is to solve this problem and answer the question. Cheryl's aim becomes 'The aim of this review is to evaluate the effectiveness of spinal bracing as compared with other treatments at reducing spinal curvature, rib hump and psychological problems'. The main difference between the review question and the aim is that the former is a question and the latter is a statement. Before Cheryl writes her objectives, she has to consider what she will need to do in order to conduct the review. Cheryl's objectives could be, for example:

- Search for papers on the effectiveness of braces and all other treatments.
- Collect data on the effectiveness of braces and all other treatments.

- Compare primary papers on the effectiveness of the treatments above.
- Compare the findings of this review with other reviews.
- Provide guidelines on the effectiveness of the different treatments for helping adolescent patients with scoliosis.

Case studies

The following case studies for Sue and Mary are introduced below.

Ⓢ Case study: intensive care nurse Sue

Sue is an experienced qualified nurse working in an intensive care unit. She has seen a number of patients who have been brought into A&E following severe car accidents and have been resuscitated. She has witnessed the grief that relatives experienced, which was exacerbated when they had not been allowed to be with their loved ones during this traumatic event. This was made worse if their relative died and they had not been present during the attempted resuscitation. Sue decided to conduct a systematic review on this subject as part of her professional development.

Ⓜ Case study: A&E nurse Mary

Mary is a newly qualified nurse working in A&E, who often sees women who have been physically abused and brought in with severe facial and body bruises. This has led her to become interested in the area of domestic violence. Her review question is: 'For women who have experienced domestic violence, how effective are advocacy programmes as compared with routine treatments on women's quality of life (as measured by a specific validated scale)?'

Mary's aim will be similar to her question, for example: 'The aim of this review is to evaluate the effectiveness of advocacy programmes as compared with other treatments on the quality of life of women victims of domestic violence'. As you can see in both the question and the aim, Mary has stated the population, the intervention, the comparative intervention and the outcomes. The next step is for her to write out her objectives. Like Cheryl, Sue and Mary need to consider all the activities they will be doing in order to conduct their systematic literature reviews, so Mary's objectives could be as follows:

- Search for papers on the effectiveness of advocacy programmes and other treatments.
- Collect data on the effectiveness of advocacy programmes and other treatments.
- Compare primary papers on the different treatments.
- Compare the findings of this review with other reviews.
- Provide guidelines for helping women victims of domestic violence.

Issues to consider when writing your problem statement, aims, objectives, review question and title

It is important when writing your review to ensure that you are always saying the same thing when writing out the title, the problem statement, the review question, the aim and objectives. A common mistake among student nurses we have taught is that they have used different terms when writing out each of the above, resulting in the title and aims being different. You will notice in the two examples in Tables 5.1 and 5.2 that the same words are used throughout.

Ⓜ **Table 5.1** Mary's example on domestic violence (quantitative review)

Problem statement	Little is known on the effectiveness of advocacy programmes as compared with other treatments on women's quality of life for women who have experienced domestic violence.
Review question	For women who have experienced domestic violence, how effective are advocacy programmes as compared with other treatments on women's quality of life?
Aim	The aim of this study is to evaluate the effectiveness of advocacy programmes as compared with other treatments on women's quality of life for women who have experienced domestic violence.
Objectives	• Search for papers on the effectiveness of advocacy programmes and other treatments • Collect data on the effectiveness of advocacy programmes and other treatments • Compare the primary papers on the different treatments • Compare the findings of this review with other reviews • Provide guidelines for helping women who have experienced domestic violence.
Title	A systematic literature review on the effectiveness of advocacy programmes, as compared with other treatments on women's quality of life, for women who have experienced domestic violence

Ⓢ **Table 5.2** Sue's example on witnessed resuscitation (qualitative review)

Problem statement	Little is known about the lived experience of patients, family members and healthcare professionals on family presence during resuscitation and/or invasive procedures.
Review question	Family presence during resuscitation and/or invasive procedures: what is the lived experience of patients, family members and healthcare professionals?
Aim	The aim of this systematic review is to evaluate the lived experience of patients, family members and healthcare professionals regarding family presence during resuscitation and/or invasive procedures.

(continued)

§ **Table 5.2** continued

Objectives	• Search for papers on the lived experience of patients, family members and healthcare professionals • Collect data on the lived experience of patients, family members and healthcare professionals • Compare the lived experiences of the different healthcare professionals • Compare the findings of this review with other reviews • Provide guidelines associated with family presence during resuscitation
Title	A systematic literature review on family presence during resuscitation and/ or invasive procedures: the lived experience of patients, family members and healthcare professionals.

Once you have done this, use the template in Practice Session 5.1 to write the problem statement, review question, aim, objectives and title for your own review.

Practice session 5.1

Write down the problem statement, review question, aim, objectives and title for your own review question in Box 5.3.

Box 5.3   Template for recording the problem statement, review question, aim, objectives and title for your review question

Problem statement

Review question

Aim

Objectives

Title

When you have filled in all the details for your own review question, read them through again to make sure that for each section you are stating the same thing. It may be worth giving it to a colleague to read to see if he or she agrees with you.

Specifying the inclusion and exclusion criteria for selecting your primary research papers

Stating your inclusion and exclusion criteria before you conduct the review is important. This section is where you describe the criteria that you will be using to include any research studies in your review. Torgerson (2003) suggests that a high-quality systematic review should have inclusion and exclusion criteria that are 'rigorously and transparently reported *a priori* (before you start the review)' (Torgerson 2003: 26). You may well ask 'Why is this necessary?' The reason is so that your search can target the papers that will answer your question and exclude any irrelevant ones. The criteria need to be explicit and applied stringently (Torgerson 2003). The criteria you select should follow from the research question, keeping in mind the PICO or PEO format. You will need to describe the types of research studies (T) you will be including, the participants, interventions, comparative groups (if any) and outcome measures. PICO now becomes PICOT. For qualitative systematic reviews use PEO (which will now become PEOT). Please note that whether you are writing a qualitative or quantitative review, all of these steps are the same with the exception that for qualitative reviews the data extraction and presentation of results are conducted a little differently from quantitative reviews. Further details on these differences can be found in Chapters 7 and 8. How to specify the inclusion and exclusion criteria for each component (PICOT or PEOT) of your review question will now be discussed.

Specifying the types of studies to be included and excluded

When selecting your primary research papers, it is important to select papers with the appropriate design for your particular review question. If you are evaluating the effectiveness of an intervention, the highest quality research designs will be RCTs or CCTs. (Please refer to the research design section in Chapter 2 to go over the different research designs if you are still uncertain about this.) You could also use other research designs that do not include a control intervention, but these will be lower on the hierarchical scale of quality of evidence (see Chapter 2).

In a Cochrane systematic review we conducted with an international team of colleagues, both RCTs and CCTs were included; we also included prospective cohort studies because we knew there were not many RCTs (Negrini et al. 2010, Negrini et al. 2015).

In the case studies, Cheryl and Mary will be seeking similar papers as they are looking at conducting quantitative reviews on the effectiveness of interventions. They have excluded case studies, because case studies are very low down on the quality of evidence scale. If there was very little information available, however, it may be worth considering the inclusion of case studies designs.

In contrast, Sue will be evaluating people's lived experiences of witnessed resuscitation and will be conducting a qualitative review. If you plan to conduct a qualitative review, you will be searching for primary qualitative papers. The specific type of qualitative paper (i.e. phenomenological, ethnographic or grounded theory among others) will depend on your specific qualitative review question. Tables 5.3, 5.4 and 5.5

illustrate how the three different examples can be presented. These can be presented in tables or in narrative format as you prefer.

Ⓒ **Table 5.3** Cheryl's example for her scoliosis review (quantitative intervention study)

Type of studies	Include	Exclude
Quantitative	Randomized controlled trials	Commentaries
	Controlled clinical trials	Review documents
	Cohort	Case studies
		Qualitative studies

Ⓜ **Table 5.4** Mary's example for her domestic violence review (quantitative intervention study)

Type of studies	Include	Exclude
Quantitative	Randomized controlled trials	Commentaries
	Controlled clinical trials	Review documents
	Cohort	Case studies
		Qualitative studies

Ⓢ **Table 5.5** Sue's example for her witnessed resuscitation review (qualitative study)

Type of studies	Include	Exclude
Qualitative	Phenomenological	Letters
	Grounded theory	Commentaries
	Descriptive	Reviews
	Ethnography	Discussion papers
		Quantitative studies

Specifying the types of participants to be included and excluded

Ⓒ To explain this process let's begin by discussing Cheryl's case study. Cheryl plans to include only children and adolescents aged 10 years of age or older when diagnosed. She makes it clear that the primary research papers she needs to find will include only those related to adolescents or children. She is also specifying that the age limit for including children will be either until they stop growing (as measured by pelvis or wrist radiographs or both) or until they are 18 years old. Cheryl needs to be specific as to the types of patients she will be excluding. She has decided to exclude any patients where scoliosis was not the primary diagnosis, such as congenital, neurological, metabolic and post-traumatic. Cheryl's example can be seen in Table 5.6.

ℭ **Table 5.6** Cheryl's case study inclusion and exclusion criteria

Review	Inclusion criteria	Exclusion criteria
Clinical population and diagnosis	*(State who the population will be and provide an operational definition)* Patients with adolescent idiopathic scoliosis (i.e. patients who develop a curve and rib hump when they are 10 years of age or older and for which there is no known cause)	*(Specify what types of diagnosis will be excluded)* Adults with idiopathic or degenerative scoliosis and adolescents with any type of secondary scoliosis (e.g. neurological, metabolic, post-traumatic)
Age	*(Provide the upper and lower age limits with a rationale)* Age 10–18 or until the end of bone growth and measured by an x-ray of the wrist or pelvis	Children under 10, adults over 18 years of age and adolescents whose bone growth has ended
Stage or severity of disease	*(In some clinical conditions it is important to know how long they have had the disease as the symptoms are likely to be more severe)* All curve types and magnitudes	Curves >50 degrees
Other factors relevant to your population group	*(Include any factors that it is important for the reader to know)* As defined by the Scoliosis Research Society (2006)	

𝕊 Let us now consider Sue's case study on witnessed resuscitation. Sue plans to include adult patients over the age of 18 years up to 60 years of age. She thinks that patients younger or older than this age range may have perceptions that are quite different. Sue needs to provide the operational definition again, which in her case is 'resuscitation or invasive procedures' as well as the setting which will be 'within a tertiary setting (hospital)'. She also specifies the type of injury 'after suffering cardiac arrest or substantial injury warranting a lifesaving intervention'.

Finally, as Sue will be looking into the perspectives of three different populations – that is the patient, the family members and the healthcare professionals – she needs to specify who these will be. Family members include spouse, partner, close friend, carer, parent, sibling, son and daughter. Healthcare professionals include any named nurse, charge nurse, nurse practitioner or sister whose role is advocating for the patient and who is part of the resuscitation team or is involved with the patient and family in the capacity of delivering a 'duty of care'. Other professionals include the consultant, specialist, doctor, surgeon, physiotherapist, social worker or occupational therapist. In Table 5.7 Sue includes three different populations to evaluate if there are differences in perceptions among them.

§ **Table 5.7** The three population criteria Sue specified for her witnessed resuscitation review

Review	Inclusion criteria	Exclusion criteria
Population 1 *Patient*	Adult patients >18 years undergoing cardiopulmonary resuscitation/invasive procedure	No children <18 years, patients undergoing chemotherapy, patients suffering from chronic illness or who have a DNAR (do not attempt resuscitation). No lay person, onlooker, hospital porter, ward clerk
Population 2 *Family members*	Spouse, partner, close friend, carer, parent, sibling, son, daughter	Bystanders, friends
Population 3 *Healthcare professionals*	Named nurse, charge nurse, nurse practitioner, sister, consultant, specialist, doctor, surgeon, physiotherapist, social worker, occupational therapist	Ward clerk, porters, housekeepers, priest

Ⓜ In Table 5.8 Mary records the population criteria for her domestic violence review.

Ⓜ **Table 5.8** The population criteria Mary specified for her domestic violence review

Review	Inclusion criteria	Exclusion criteria
Population	Women	Men, children and teenagers
	Adults >18 years	Women in lesbian relationships
	Experiencing or have experienced domestic violence in the past	Women with disabilities Pregnant women

In summary, when describing the inclusion and exclusion criteria for your population(s), it is important that you clearly state who the population(s) will be, specify their diagnosis, the severity and duration of the disease, who will be included as well as any other relevant factors as discussed above.

Practice session 5.2

Use the template in Box 5.4 for writing down the population criteria for your own review.

Box 5.4 Template for recording your own population criteria		
Review	*Inclusion criteria*	*Exclusion criteria*
Clinical population	*(State who the population will be and provide an operational definition)*	
Diagnosis	*(State and define the diagnosis)*	
Age	*(Provide the upper and lower age limits with a rationale)*	
Stage or severity of disease	*(In some clinical conditions, it is important to know how long patients have had the disease as the symptoms are likely to be more severe)*	
Other factors relevant to your population group	*(These can include any other factors that you think are important to include)*	

Specifying the interventions (or exposure) to be included and excluded

You could start this section by first describing the interventions you plan to evaluate for your review. Cheryl's example is shown in Table 5.9.

[M] With regards to Mary's review on domestic violence, she provides a brief explanation of what is meant by 'community advocacy programmes' and then states which different types of programmes she will be including. In this section it would also be

Ⓒ **Table 5.9** Cheryl's intervention criteria

Intervention	Inclusion criteria	Exclusion criteria
Intervention	All types of rigid, semi-rigid and elastic braces, worn for a specific number of hours, for a specific number of years	Electrotherapy Traction Exercise only
Comparative intervention	All possible control interventions and comparisons were included	None

useful for her to state clearly whether the papers she is planning to use will include all types of programmes or only those with particular characteristics, for example only those that are run by women who have themselves experienced domestic violence and not those run only by healthcare professionals. One way of presenting the inclusion and exclusion criteria for Mary's review on domestic violence is shown in Table 5.10.

Ⓜ **Table 5.10** Mary's intervention criteria

Intervention	Inclusion criteria	Exclusion criteria
Intervention	Advocacy (conducted within or outside of health setting) Community programmes (need to include a clear definition of these)	Not formal cognitive–behavioural therapy
Comparative intervention	Usual general practitioner (GP) treatment (usually this means no treatment for domestic violence)	Other interventions Alternative therapies

Another point to consider is whether or not you are planning to include interventions carried out all over the world or just in the UK. The Cochrane Collaboration (2009) recommends finding all available studies from all over the world, but if your specific review question relates to treatment methods conducted within the UK, it is best to explain this and provide a rationale. Sue's inclusion and exclusion criteria for her review on witnessed resuscitation are shown in Table 5.11; her inclusion criteria are very comprehensive.

Ⓢ **Table 5.11** Sue's inclusion and exclusion criteria for her exposure criteria

	Inclusion criteria	Exclusion criteria
Exposure Witnessed cardiopulmonary resuscitation after patient suffers a cardiac arrest OR Invasive procedures performed while undergoing resuscitation or as a lifesaving measure	Tertiary setting, such as hospital intensive care unit (ICU), paediatric intensive care unit (PICU), maternity departments, coronary care unit (CCU), high dependency unit (HDU), accident and emergency departments (A&E) Patient's home, ambulance or community setting	Hospice setting Rehabilitation establishment

Specifying the comparative interventions to be included and excluded

The comparative intervention needs to be specified if you are using the PICO format but not if you plan to use the PEO format. If you have a comparative intervention, you need to state the inclusion and exclusion criteria for the comparative intervention(s) you will be including within your review. The comparative interventions for the two quantitative studies can be seen in Tables 5.9 and 5.10.

Ⓢ **Table 5.12** Sue's criteria for considering studies in her review based on the PEO structure

Outcomes	Inclusion criteria	Exclusion criteria
Psychological issues, experience, perception, views, feelings	Experiences, perceptions, views from all members of the population groups toward resuscitation and invasive procedures	Physical effects: insomnia, tachycardia, guilt

Ⓜ **Table 5.13** Mary's criteria for considering studies in her review based on the PICO structure

Outcomes	Inclusion criteria	Exclusion criteria
Quantitative	Validated quality of life (QOL) scales (need to specify which ones)	Qualitative experiences

Specifying the outcomes to be included and excluded

By outcome measures we are usually referring to measurable outcomes or clinical changes in health (Khan et al. 2003). Outcomes include body structures and functions like pain and fatigue, activities as in functional abilities and participation or quality of life questionnaires as seen in Box 5.5.

Box 5.5   Types of outcome measures

You will need to state what type of outcome measures will be included; examples are listed below.

- Body structures and functions – weight, pain, fatigue.
- Activities – functional abilities, dexterity.
- Participation – physical independence, quality of life.
- Process measures – compliance, strength.
- Others – rates of domestic violence.
- If it is a qualitative review – experiences of subjects.

Box 5.6 shows how Cheryl could write out her outcome measures.

Practical Tip

Note that it is not enough to state that you will be measuring 'quality of life'. You also need to add what standardized assessment tools or validated measuring instruments will be included. It is pointless including scales that are not reliable and/or validated as their results might not be accurate.

Ⓒ Box 5.6   Cheryl's outcome measures

Progression of scoliosis as measured by:

- the Cobb angle in degrees (the Cobb angle was devised by a surgeon (John Cobb) and measures the curvature of the spine)
- number of patients who have progressed by more than five degrees Cobb.

Quality of life and disability as measured by:

- specific validated quality of life questionnaires such as SRS-22 (Asher et al. 2003), SF-36 (Lai et al. 2006), and BSSK (Weiss et al. 2006).

Back pain as measured by:

- validated visual analogue scales (visual analogue scales provide a simple technique for measuring subjective experience: McCormack et al. 1988)
- use of medication
- adverse effects as measured in the identified papers will be reported.

In Sue's example the 'outcomes' she will be looking at are the experiences, views or perceptions of her three different populations (Table 5.12). Mary's intervention review question (Table 5.13) is similar to Cheryl's intervention review question.

Useful resources associated with nursing outcomes

The Collaborative Alliance for Nursing Outcomes (CALNOC):
  http://www.calnoc.org/

International Council for Nursing 'Nursing sensitive outcome indicators':
  http://www.icn.ch/images/stories/documents/publications/fact_sheets/15c_
  FS-Nursing_Sensitive_Outcome_Indicators.pdf

Finally we will discuss Fay's example on CAUTI. The protocol for Fay's literature review was shown in Chapter 3. In the section below we have included Fay's own introduction to this section of her dissertation as it provides a good example.

F Fay's case study on CAUTI

Fay is a fictitious name for a student nurse studying the Bachelor of Nursing Science a number of years ago, as previously mentioned on page 37. Fay undertook a systematic review and kindly gave permission for us to use her research question, as also discussed in Chapter 3 where we reproduced her protocol. We believe her work significantly helps to illustrate key aspects of the systematic review. Although we acknowledge that her thesis requires updating we are also of the opinion that her work offers sound insights into undertaking a review. She had encountered many patients with CAUTIs both during her placements in hospital as well as in her placements in the community and was a little confused by the recommendations for catheter insertion at the time. Her area of interest was UTIs. The aim of her review was to evaluate the existing guidelines (back in 2008) that promoted the practice of *not* using antiseptics at catheter insertion. So her research question was 'In patients requiring urinary catheterisation is sterile catheter insertion more effective than non-sterile insertion at reducing the incidence of catheter associated urinary tract infection (CAUTI)?' (As Fay completed her dissertation in 2008 please accept our apologies if any guidelines/recommendations are now outdated or have been changed. We have also not included all Fay's references within the book's reference list as these are for purely illustrative purposes only.)

Fay's introduction to her chapter on specifying her inclusion and exclusion criteria

The following is an extract from Fay's introduction to her chapter on specifying her inclusion and exclusion criteria.

The criteria for the selection of studies to be included in a review need to be defined ahead of the selection process in order to avoid selection bias (Khan et al. 2003, pg 29). The components of the structured question are used to generate a list of selection criteria. Using the PICO framework facilitates the process. The study types or designs are identified after considering their likely suitability at answering the review question and their level on the evidence hierarchy, while also bearing in mind the probable abundance or scarcity of the relevant studies. Torgerson (2003, pg 27–28) recommends a rapid scope of the literature early in the planning stage to establish how plentiful relevant studies are; this also serves to identify existing reviews, however, Torgerson also warns that this could be a source of bias in the review.

Commentary on Fay's inclusion and exclusion criteria

For ease of use the inclusion and exclusion criteria for Fay's case study have been copied into Table 5.14. Please note that on the left hand side of the table is what Fay actually wrote in her real dissertation and to the right is our commentary.

Table 5.14 Example of student nurse Fay's inclusion and exclusion criteria

	Inclusion	Exclusion	Commentary on Fay's criteria
Types of studies T	Comparative studies: randomised controlled trials; prospective clinical control trials; cohort studies with a control group; case study with a control group, any prospective studies with a control group	Single group studies; cohort studies without a control; qualitative studies	The best study designs to answer review questions regarding the effectiveness of an intervention are comparative studies; these studies compare the effect of the intervention on an outcome in the study group with the same outcome in the control group (who are not exposed to the intervention being assessed). Such studies feature high on the hierarchy of evidence when allocation to the two groups is randomized and concealed (RCTs); bias is avoided since any confounding variables are equally distributed between the two groups (Craig and Smyth 2007: 89–92). However, following a rapid scope of the literature, it was evident that studies relevant to the review question were unlikely to be numerous; therefore it was deemed necessary that other designs (shown on the left) which are not considered as sound as RCTs, were also included. In other words Fay has included most quantitative study designs that were prospective and with a control group, even case studies as otherwise she risked not finding enough studies for her review.
P	Male or female patients undergoing urinary catheterisation performed by a healthcare worker Short term/long term indwelling or intermittent catheterisation Setting: hospital, rehabilitation unit or nursing home	Intermittent self-catheterisation, Supra-pubic catheterisation, pre-existing urinary tract infection, urological surgery, patients on antibiotics	Both male and female patients were included as Fay wanted to know the outcomes for both genders. She has also specified that this needed to be done by a health worker. Why do you think she is stating this? She is stating this so as to try and make her study as free from error as possible and make the group she is including as similar as possible. If the patient or a family member performed the procedure this may have introduced more bacteria than a healthcare worker. Patients who required and underwent urinary catheterization, whether indwelling (short term or long term) or intermittent, and which was performed by a healthcarer were included in the review. However, patients who underwent intermittent self-catheterization were excluded along with those having pre-existing urinary tract infections, those who had undergone urological surgery and those who were on antibiotics.

I	Sterile urethral catheterisation	The interventions under investigation were the sterile or aseptic catheter insertion technique and the specific steps involved in the process, namely hand washing, sterile gloves and gowns, antiseptic meatal cleansing and use of antiseptic lubricating gel.
C	Other forms of catheterisation • Non-sterile urethral catheterisation • Hand washing is omitted or modified and / or • No sterile gloves are used and / or • No sterile gowns are used and / or • No antiseptic meatal cleansing and /or • Lubricating gel used contains no antiseptic	Non-sterile or clean catheter insertion techniques were the comparisons or controls examined; these included insertion techniques or their component steps that did not use antiseptics or sterile equipment as used in the sterile technique. Also included were insertion techniques where one or more of the specific steps of the sterile approach were either omitted or modified and/or where any of the following processes mentioned in the inclusion criteria for the comparative intervention seen on the left occurred.
O	Any other outcomes CAUTI confirmed by significant bacteriuria or clinical symptoms or urethral colony counts	The rate of incidence of CAUTI was considered as the outcome measure. CAUTI was identified as established by the presence of its clinical symptoms and/or the presence of significant bacteriuria. Significant bacteriuria was defined as 100,000 CFU/ml and was considered to be more reliable at diagnosing CAUTI since the latter may be asymptomatic. It was assumed that CAUTI which could, safely, be attributed directly to catheter insertion would occur within the first few days following insertion and hence urine samples showing significant bacteriuria within this period would be most reliable.

Practice session 5.3

For your own review question, select the appropriate template (PICO or PEO) and write out the inclusion and exclusion criteria for all the PICO (Box 5.7) or PEO (Box 5.8) components

Box 5.7   PICO template to use for your own inclusion and exclusion criteria

	Inclusion criteria	Exclusion criteria
Population		
Intervention		
Comparative groups		
Outcome		
Type of studies		

Box 5.8   PEO template to use for your own inclusion and exclusion criteria

	Inclusion criteria	Exclusion criteria
Population		
Exposure		
Outcome		
Type of studies		

Key points

- A problem statement is a simple statement of 'what is'.
- The review question follows from the problem statement.
- The 'aim' of a project is to solve the problem and answer the review question.
- The 'objective' is usually more specific than the aim.
- The objectives state what the researcher is going to do.
- Your aims and objectives need to be written clearly and concisely.
- Always make sure you can identify the PICO or PEO elements within them.
- When writing your objectives think of what it is you will actually be doing.
- Ensure that your aims, objectives, research question and title are all saying the same thing. The best way of doing this is to use virtually the same words for all four.

- A high-quality systematic literature review should have inclusion and exclusion criteria that are reported before the review is conducted.

- It is important that your search can target the papers that will answer your question and exclude any irrelevant ones.

- The inclusion and exclusion criteria for your review need to be explicit and applied stringently.

Summary

This chapter discussed the meanings of and differences between a problem statement, a review question, aims and objectives. Methods of specifying the inclusion and exclusion criteria for the types of studies, the population(s), intervention, comparative intervention(s) or exposures and outcome measures were discussed and examples provided for quantitative and qualitative review questions. Templates were provided to help you write out your own problem statement, aims and objectives and your inclusion and exclusion criteria.

Question and Answer (Q&A)

(Q) What are the pitfalls that result from not having identified clear inclusion and exclusion criteria?

(A) Articulating clear inclusion and exclusion criteria enables you to identify, locate and choose the most relevant articles for review. Having unclear inclusion and exclusion criteria has the potential to impact on the quality and outcomes of the final review. It also makes sure that the process you use to select your papers for inclusion/exclusion within your review is always based on the same criteria. If the criteria are not very clear then you may find that you will select some papers based on some criteria and you will select other papers based on some unwritten criteria; for instance if you found a paper written by a famous professor that was in a very similar area but did not strictly meet all your inclusion criteria, then you might be tempted to include it in your review.

6
Conducting a comprehensive and systematic literature search

Overview

- Importance of undertaking a comprehensive and systematic search
- Aims of undertaking a comprehensive and systematic search
- Key factors to be considered when undertaking a comprehensive search
- Steps involved in converting your review question into a comprehensive search strategy

Importance of undertaking a comprehensive and systematic search

When you conduct a systematic review, it is important that you try to retrieve all studies (or as many as possible) relating to the specific question that your review is addressing. This means searching as widely as possible from a whole range of sources. Although you may eventually exclude some papers (if they do not meet all your inclusion criteria) it is important that all the relevant studies are found and considered to ensure that your sample (all the studies you include) is as unbiased as possible. It is usually necessary to search a wide variety of databases and internet search engines as well as hand searching, which 'involves a manual page-by-page examination of the entire contents of a journal issue to identify all eligible reports of trials, whether they appear in articles, abstracts, news columns, editorials, letters or other text' (Higgins and Deeks 2009).

Practical Tip

If you are unfamiliar with searching for evidence on the internet and using different databases, before actually starting your comprehensive literature search it might be useful to contact your library and see if they have a course on 'Literature searching' for healthcare studies. This could save you a great amount of time in the long term. Additionally you could also speak to the librarian to see if they could support you in other ways.

Aims of undertaking a comprehensive and systematic search

The aim of the search is to generate a comprehensive list of primary studies, both published and unpublished, that may be suitable for answering the proposed research question. The validity (truthfulness) of the review is directly related to the thoroughness of the search and its ability to identify all the relevant studies (Centre for Reviews and Dissemination 2008). Conducting a comprehensive literature search helps to identify current knowledge with regard to relevant concepts and contexts and what is known and unknown in a particular field (Petticrew and Roberts 2006).

A comprehensive search strategy underlies the quality of the literature search, which in turn underlies the quality of the findings for the systematic review (Higgins and Green 2011). Any conclusions made following the review are only as good as the range and quality of the literature obtained.

It is important to search widely and thoroughly because not all research is published in journals. Additionally, not all the research published in journals is indexed in major databases and may not be easily retrievable (Bruce et al. 2008). Other reasons for searching widely include the fact that there may be a long wait before publication. Publication gaps after conference presentations are common because it takes authors a considerable amount of time to write up their findings, submit them, get them reviewed and then amended as necessary. Discovering a conference paper before publication could be important as it will provide some, although limited, information.

Problems with searching include publication and language bias (Dickersin et al. 1987). Publication bias means that positive results tend to be published more frequently than negative results in journals (Bruce et al. 2008). Language bias refers to the fact that positive results are more likely to be published in English. Egger et al. (1997) found that researchers who obtained statistically significant results in RCTs were more likely to publish in an English-language journal. Researchers and students are more likely to read research in their own language.

Bias may also relate to the geographical coverage of journals and databases. Some journals and databases tend to publish articles originating primarily from certain countries. The MEDLINE database, for example, includes approximately 10 million references, more than half (62 per cent) of which originate from the United States alone (Bruce et al. 2008).

Key factors to be considered when undertaking a comprehensive search

A number of key factors should be considered when undertaking a search for relevant articles, including the following.

- Reading reference lists will identify source ideas and concepts that highlight the design of studies. Similarly looking at the contents pages of journals is also a good way of identifying ideas and potential knowledge gaps.

- Hand searching may help to avoid possible bias in 'keyword' search systems. Keyword search systems like MEDLINE help reviewers to identify published studies more easily. However, Armstrong et al. state:

Information technology and the processes associated with indexing are not infallible. Studies may not be correctly marked by study design which may mean they are missed in the electronic searching process. Hand searching for evidence of intervention effectiveness has therefore become a recognized tool in the systematic review process.

(Armstrong et al. 2005: 388)

- Accessing 'grey' literature, for example conference proceedings and PhD theses, will provide smaller and unpublished studies that may still be robust enough to provide valuable information.

- Getting in touch with authors of key articles may lead to them providing access to some of their important but unpublished work.

- Talking to colleagues about who are the experts in the area is another good way of identifying potential sources of work.

Steps involved in converting your review question into a comprehensive search strategy

There are a number of steps involved in converting the review question into a search strategy. The first step is to refer back to the keywords that will form the basis of the search. Timmins and McCabe (2005: 44) stated that 'The use of appropriate keywords is the cornerstone of an effective search'. It is possible to conduct searches using both index terms and free text searching. Index terms include terms used by electronic databases, which may not precisely match the terms in the research question, for example the Medical Subject Headings (MeSH) database in MEDLINE. To ensure that a search is comprehensive and both sensitive and specific, free text searching, also known as 'natural language' or language we use daily, should be used in addition to or instead of index term searching (Lahlafi 2007). This section provides an overview of all the steps involved in conducting a comprehensive search for a systematic literature review in nursing practice. This includes a discussion of the whole process and will be illustrated by two of the case studies introduced in previous chapters.

Step 1: write out the research question and identify the component parts

As mentioned in Chapter 2, the first step is to write out the research question and identify the PICO (population, intervention, comparative intervention, outcomes) or PEO (population, exposure, outcomes) components. Templates are provided for both the PICO and PEO types of questions below. Referring back to two of the case studies (Mary and Cheryl), these can be written out as shown in Tables 6.1 and 6.2.

Table 6.1 Key components of Mary's intervention research question on domestic violence based on the PICO structure

P	I	C	O
Women who have experienced domestic violence	Advocacy programmes	General practice or routine treatment	Quantitative quality of life (measured by the SF-36 scale)

Table 6.2 Key components of Cheryl's intervention research question on adolescent idiopathic scoliosis based on the PICO structure

P	I	C	O
Patients with adolescent idiopathic scoliosis	how effective is spinal bracing	as compared with other treatments	at reducing spinal curvature, rib hump and psychological problems?

Practice session 6.1

Once you have read Mary and Cheryl's examples, use one of the empty templates below based on the PICO and PEO structures to write out the components of your own review question (Boxes 6.1 and 6.2). You could add another column T if you wish to include the type of studies you will be including.

Box 6.1   PICO template to use for your own review question

P	I	C	O

Step 2: identify any synonyms

The second step is to identify any synonyms (words that mean the same thing) for all the component parts (P, I, C, O or P, E, O) of the review question. For example, other terms for 'scoliosis' are 'curvature of the spine', or 'spinal deformity'. It is essential to understand that any search needs to be both sensitive and specific. Sensitivity (in this context) refers to a search that picks up all the research articles that are potentially relevant. Specificity refers to a search that selects only those research articles that are directly relevant.

It is important to identify all the synonyms relating to the question and then to combine them using specific words called Boolean operators: these are words used in

Box 6.2 PEO template to use for your own review question

P	*E*	*O*

searches to combine different keywords or phrases. A list of the most common operators include the following.

- OR – finds citations containing either of the specified keywords or phrases (sensitivity).
- AND – finds citations containing all of the specified keywords or phrases (specificity).
- NOT – excludes citations containing specified keywords or phrases.

The various steps will be identified using the case studies involving Mary and Cheryl.

M *Mary's case study: identifying synonyms and combining keywords*

Mary is researching domestic violence and needs to identify synonyms for all the PICO components of her research question (Table 6.1). She is having difficulty thinking of synonyms, so she decides to use a thesaurus. To help her in this task she uses a template (Table 6.3). This template has a column for each letter of PICO (these can also be called strings) and a row for each synonym.

Using this type of template enables Mary to combine all the related terms of her question to try to obtain as many relevant articles as possible. It also optimizes the sensitivity and specificity of her search. In order to explain this further, let's refer back to her question above. If we start with the population column P, Mary first needs to find synonyms for 'women who have experienced domestic violence'. Synonyms for this could include 'wife abuse', 'partner abuse', 'battered women' and 'spouse abuse'. In Table 6.4, Mary first creates a list under the heading of Patient/condition with each synonym in a new row and numbers them from 1 to 9 (there just happen to be nine in this particular case).

The numbers represent the order or the individual steps of how the words will be typed into the search database (for example EBSCO or CINAHL) and have been

Table 6.3 This is the empty template used by Mary to identify the synonyms for her review question. Try and help her combine her keywords

Column terms combined with	Patient/condi-tion AND	Intervention AND	Comparative intervention AND	Outcomes AND
OR				
OR				
OR				
OR				

Table 6.4 Mary's completed template used to identify the synonyms for her review question and help her combine her keywords

Column terms combined with	Patient/condition AND	Intervention AND	Comparative inter-vention AND	Outcomes AND
OR	1 Domestic violence	11 Treatment	21 General practice	28 Women's quality of life
OR	2 Wife abuse	12 Group support	22 GP	
OR	3 Partner abuse	13 Individual support	23 Routine treatment	
OR	4 Battered women	14 Advocacy programme	24 Doctor	
OR	6 Spouse abuse	16 Counselling	26 Physician	
OR	6 Rape	16 Community	26 Surgery	
OR	7 Sexual abuse	17 Therapy		
OR	8 Coercion	18 Support		
OR	9 Murder	19 Advocacy		
	10 Combine 1–9 using 'OR'	20 Combine 11–19 using 'OR'	27 Combine 21–26 using 'OR'	28

The last step is to combine steps 10+20+27+28 together using the term 'AND'

included to help you understand how this process is conducted. This is repeated for the intervention 'I' (steps 11–19), the comparative intervention 'C' (steps 21–26) and the outcomes 'O' (step 28). When all the words in each of the four columns have been combined with 'OR', all the synonyms for P, I, C and O are combined using the Boolean term 'AND'. Thus the final part of the search strategy is to combine steps 10+20+27+28 together using the Boolean term 'AND'. I know this sounds very complicated but once you have followed the three examples below, the process should be much clearer.

Step 3: identify truncations and abbreviations

Once you have identified your synonyms, the third step is to identify any truncations or abbreviations. The symbol $ is a shortcut termed 'truncation' and identifies variations of a word. What this means is if Mary, for example, searched using the word 'therapy', the search would only look for the word 'therapy' and leave out anything like therapeutic, therapist, therapists, etc. In some databases you may find that the truncation is indicated with a star * at the end of the word. Please make sure that you read all the relevant information specific to the database before you use it to ensure that you are using the correct truncation sign.

Practical Tip

If in any doubt consult with a librarian.

Mary was finding this part a little hard so she looked at other reviews on a similar topic and also used a hard copy thesaurus (these tend to be much more comprehensive than online ones) and a dictionary to help her. Going back to Mary's example, her truncations ($ dollar sign) can be seen in Table 6.5. If you find this part quite hard there is no need to worry. This step is not absolutely necessary because you can also conduct the search using the full terms: it will just take a bit longer.

Sometimes it is also necessary to identify abbreviations that are commonly used. For example, the intervention 'cognitive–behavioural therapy' is frequently found as CBT in the literature.

Table 6.5 An example of how Mary could identify truncations for her key terms

Column terms combined with	Patient/condition AND	Intervention AND	Comparative intervention AND	Outcomes AND
OR	1 Domestic violence	11 Treat$	21 General practice	28 Women's quality of life
OR	2 Wife abuse	12 Group support	22 GP	
OR	3 Partner abuse	13 Individual support	23 Routine treatment	
OR	4 Battered wom$	14 Advocacy program$	24 Doctor$	
OR	6 Spouse abuse	16 Counsel$	26 Physician$	
OR	6 Rape	16 Community	26 Surger$	
OR	7 Sexual abuse	17 Therap$		
OR	8 Coerc$	18 Support		
OR	9 Murder	19 Advocacy		
	10 Combine 1–9 using 'OR'	20 Combine 11–19 using 'OR'	27 Combine 21–26 using 'OR'	28

The last step is to combine steps 10+20+27+28 together using the term 'AND'

ℂ *Cheryl's case study: identifying synonyms*

As with Mary's case study, Cheryl begins by identifying the key components of her review question (Table 6.2) and then starts identifying the synonyms to her keywords.

Cheryl's population group are patients with adolescent idiopathic scoliosis. She writes this under the population heading (column) and numbers it 1. What other synonyms are there for AIS? She could use the terms 'spinal deformity' (2), 'spinal curvature' (3), 'lateral curvature' (4), 'crooked spine' (6), 'rib hump' (6) and 'poor posture' (7), which now all need to be numbered in sequence from 2 to 7.

Cheryl now needs to combine all the synonyms using the Boolean operator 'OR' (Table 6.6). This simply means that she is asking the search engine to search for any papers that have as a population group any of the synonyms listed. So this will be step 8 and can be written as [[combine 1–7 using 'OR']]. In other words she is trying to make her search as sensitive as possible. The Boolean operator 'OR' finds citations containing any of the specified keywords, phrases or synonyms (sensitivity).

Cheryl's next step is to repeat this process for the intervention, comparative interventions and outcomes columns on the template. The word 'brace' under the intervention heading will now be step 9, the word 'rigid brace' will now be step 10, 'semi-rigid brace' step 11, 'soft brace' step 12 and 'spinal orthosis' step 13. Cheryl cannot think of any more synonyms and cannot find any more in the thesaurus, so she now needs to let the search engine know that she would like to look for any of the listed synonyms for the word 'brace'. Cheryl will now write this as follows: step 16 [[combine 9–16 using 'OR']] and will write them in the intervention column below (Table 6.6, see page 111 for Cheryl's full search strategy list).

Cheryl continues doing this for the comparative intervention column and the outcomes. The last step is for her to combine all the 'OR' combinations for each column (8+16+24+33) using the Boolean operator 'AND', which will find citations containing all of the specified keywords or phrases (specificity). To summarize, this will enable Cheryl to make her search as sensitive and specific as possible in order to enable her to find as many relevant citations as possible to answer her review question.

Table 6.6 Template used by Cheryl to start identifying keyword synonyms

Column terms combined with	Patient/ condition AND	Intervention AND	Comparative inter- vention AND	Outcomes AND
OR	1 Patients with adolescent idiopathic scoliosis (AIS)			
OR	2 Spinal deformity			
OR	3 Spinal curvature			
OR	4 Lateral curvature			
OR	6 Crooked spine			
OR	6 Rib hump			
OR	7 Poor posture			
	8 Combine 1–7 using 'OR'			

Practice session 6.2

Now that we have discussed two examples, try to identify the synonyms and truncations for the review question you developed in Chapter 2 and then try to combine the keywords by using one of the templates provided. There are templates for both PICO and PEO formats in Boxes 6.3 and 6.4

Box 6.3   PICO template to use for your own review question to identify synonyms and combine keywords

Column terms combined with	Patient/ condition AND	Intervention AND	Comparative intervention AND	Outcomes AND
OR				
OR				
OR				
OR				

Box 6.4   PEO template to use for your own review question to identify synonyms and combine keywords

Column terms combined with	Patient/ condition AND	Exposure AND	Outcomes AND
OR			
OR			
OR			
OR			

Step 4: develop a search strategy string

The fourth step is to develop a search strategy string (i.e. a list of words) to input into the different databases. Keywords and synonyms need to be 'translated' or 'tweaked' to develop a search strategy list. The following list shows exactly which words Mary will be typing into a specific database (for example EBSCO or CINAHL or MEDLINE) to conduct her search and the order and combinations of how she will type them in. Following on from the template above, Mary first types the words from 1 to 9 individually into the database search engine. Once she has done this she will need to combine them using the word 'OR' (line 10). This is repeated for the remaining columns – intervention I (20), comparative intervention C (27) and outcomes column O (28). Once she has done this, all the PICO synonyms need to be combined using the term 'AND', which means she will need to combine the numbers 10, 20, 27 and 28. Mary's sequence for doing this is shown below.

M

1   Domestic violence
2   Wife abuse
3   Partner abuse
4   Battered women
5   Spouse abuse
6   Rape
7   Sexual abuse
8   Coercion
9   Murder
10 1 OR 2 OR 3 OR 4 OR 6 OR 5 OR 7 OR 8 OR 9 (Mary has combined terms using 'OR')
11 Treatment
12 Group support
13 Individual support
14 Advocacy programme
15 Counselling
16 Community
17 Therapy
18 Support
19 Advocacy
20 11 OR 12 OR 13 OR 14 OR 15 OR 16 OR 17 OR 18 OR 19 (Mary has combined terms using 'OR')
21 General practice
22 GP
23 Routine treatment
24 Doctor
25 Physician
26 Surgery
27 21 OR 22 OR 23 OR 24 OR 25 OR 26 (Mary has combined terms using 'OR')
28 Quality of life
29 10 AND 20 AND 27 AND 28 (Mary has combined the terms using 'AND').

It is preferable to apply limits at the final stage of the literature search. Limits can include restricting the search to English-language articles, human studies, research articles and possibly specifying a date range (you will need to provide a rationale for this, it shouldn't just be arbitrary). For example, if there had been a significant change in advocacy programmes since 1990, it would be wise to limit the search strategy to articles written after this date. Different limits are available in different databases. If limiting a search to English-language articles only, it is important to acknowledge that a language bias has been introduced into the search as you may have left out potentially important and relevant articles written in other languages.

Cheryl's strategy list example can be found below.

ℂ

1   Patients with adolescent idiopathic scoliosis
2   Spinal deformity
3   Spinal curvature
4   Lateral curvature
5   Crooked spine
6   Rib hump
7   Poor posture
8   Combine 1–7 using 'OR'
9   Brace$
10   Rigid brace$
11   Semi-rigid brace$
12   Soft brace$
13   Spinal orthosis
14   Orthopaedic device$
15   Orthopaedic equipment
16   Combine 9–16 using 'OR'
17   Exercise$
18   Brace$
19   Semi-rigid brace$
20   Rigid brace$
21   Electrical stimulation
22   Orthopaedic devices
23   Orthopaedic equipment
24   Combine 17–23 using 'OR'
25   Spinal curvature$
26   Rib hump$
27   Posture$
28   Back shape
29   Self-esteem
30   Self-confidence
31   Quality of life
32   Pain
33   Combine 26–32 using 'OR'
34   Combine 8 AND 16 AND 24 AND 33.

Practical Tip

You may want to consider using internet language translation services to help you check the titles, abstracts and other article details written in a foreign language.

Practice session 6.3

With your own review question in mind, use the template in Box 6.5 to translate all the keywords and synonyms into a search strategy list like the ones developed by Mary and Cheryl.

Box 6.5   Template to use for translating your review question keywords into a search strategy list

```
1
2
3
4
6
6
7
8
9
10
11
12
13
14
16
16
17
18
19
20
21
22
23
24
26
26
27
28
29
30
```

Step 5: undertake a comprehensive search using all possible sources of information

The fifth step, having completed your search strategy string, is to undertake a comprehensive search, using databases and all other sources of information that are most relevant to your review question. Sources of information fall into several categories including online general databases, specialist databases, journal articles, grey literature, subject gateways, conference papers and proceedings, dissertation abstracts, contacting experts (clinical and non-clinical) and books. Below is a brief description of each type of information source together with its weblink.

General databases

Online databases include general databases like CINAHL, MEDLINE and AMED. An excellent publication called 'Finding studies for systematic reviews: a checklist for researchers' is available on the Centre for Reviews and Dissemination website at http://www.york.ac.uk/crd/. This website includes a comprehensive list of the websites and other sources of information a reviewer should search when conducting a comprehensive search. Some online health databases are listed in Box 6.6.

Box 6.6   Websites for some online health databases

- MEDLINE: this is the main source for bibliographic coverage of biomedical literature; it covers 4600 journals from 1960 to the present (www.nlm.nih.gov/bsd/pmresources. html).
- CINAHL: the Cumulative Index to Nursing and Allied Health Literature is a comprehensive and authoritative resource for the professional literature of nursing, allied health, biomedicine and healthcare (www.ebscohost.com/cinahl).
- PsycINFO: The American Psychological Association's PsycINFO database records professional and academic literature in psychology and related disciplines, including medicine, psychiatry, nursing, sociology, pharmacology, physiology and linguistics (www.apa.org/pubs/databases/psycinfo/index.aspx).
- AMED: the Allied and Complementary Medicine Database covers a selection of journals related to physiotherapy, occupational therapy, palliative care and complementary medicine (https://www.ebscohost.com/academic/AMED-The-Allied-and-Complementary-Medicine-Database).
- ASSIA: the Applied Social Sciences Index and Abstracts website provides a comprehensive source of social science and health information for the practical and academic professional (www.csa.com/factsheets/assia-set-c.php).
- REHABDATA: the National Rehabilitation Information Center (NARIC) produces the REHABDATA database, providing information on physical, mental and psychiatric disabilities, independent living, vocational rehabilitation, special education, employment and assistive technology (http://www.naric.com/?q=en/home).

Evidence-Based Medicine Reviews (EBMR): this contains a number of links, including Cochrane Database of Systematic Reviews (CDSR), Database of Abstracts of Reviews of Effectiveness (DARE), American College of Physicians (ACP) Journal Club and Cochrane Controlled Trials Register (CCTR) (www.ovid.com/site/catalog/DataBase/904.jsp).

Specialist databases

There are many online specialist databases covering particular medical specialties. For example, the National Cancer Institute website can be found at http://www.cancer.gov/publications/pdq.

Journal articles

Journal articles are primary sources. These are the most up-to-date sources of peer-reviewed journals and information on advances and developments in treatment or care (most of the searches above will direct you to primary research papers).

Grey literature

Grey literature or non-journal literature refers to any unpublished sources of evidence. Most of the searches above focus on journal literature, but there are high rates of non-publication of research papers and many PhD theses are not published, therefore it is essential to search the grey literature. Grey literature also refers to published abstracts, conference proceedings, policy documents, newsletters and other unpublished written material. OpenGrey (System for Information on Grey Literature) is an open access website (www.opengrey.eu/) that has up to 700,000 bibliographical references of grey literature (paper) produced in Europe. OpenGrey covers science, technology, biomedical science, economics, social science and humanities.

Subject gateways

Subject gateways provide access to reliable and up-to-date web resources for all subjects, which have been carefully chosen and quality checked by experts in their field. Subject gateways are also called subject guides, subject directories and subject portals. They allow you to browse subject lists of good quality and evaluated subject resources. Some of the more important nursing and general health-related subject gateways are listed in Box 6.7.

Box 6.7   Websites for some nursing and general health-related subject gateways

- Nursing Portal: this is a gateway to the world of nursing (www.nursing-portal.com).
- MentalHelp.net: this website promotes mental health and wellness (www.mentalhelp.net).
- National Library for Health: the UK NHS Evidence website includes a national health library and information service (https://www.evidence.nhs.uk/).
- SearchMedica: this is an open access medical search engine (www.searchmedica.co.uk).
- Social Care Online: this promotes better knowledge for better practice (www.scie-socialcareonline.org.uk).
- Google and Google Scholar: two of the best known general purpose search engines (www.google.co.uk and scholar.google.co.uk).

Conference papers and proceedings

Conference papers and proceedings include the ISI proceedings: science and technology edition. Contains details of approximately 10,000 conferences per year (http://wok.mimas.ac.uk/).

Dissertation abstracts

Dissertation abstracts can be found at http://www.proquest.com/products-services/dissertations/.

Contacting experts (clinical and non-clinical)

The easiest way to contact experts and clinical and non-clinical specialists in your field of study is to Google their name to find a research paper that they have written. Most papers include the email address of the authors.

Books

Books are useful secondary sources for identifying 'stable' sources of information and developing your background knowledge of a research problem. Information in books can be rather old. From the time the book is first written and then published, several years may have gone by.

Step 6: save your searches

The final step is to record and save any searches as well as the results of the searches in an electronic format, so that all the necessary information will be available and easily accessible when it comes to writing up the review. The search strategy, including the database, the title of the article, the abstract, the host, for example OVID or EBSCO, and the date should be logged (see example in Box 6.8). As much detail as possible should be recorded to enable a colleague or otherwise to replicate the review

---

Box 6.8   Template example of how you could document your first search

Database	Dates covered	Date searched	Hits	Full record/titles and abstracts	Notes
MEDLINE (EBSCO host)	1990–2012	20/03/12	23	(Titles of the articles could be included here)	(You may want to give your search strategy a name, for example 'Medline1' just in case you need to run the search again sometime in the future)

if needed. This makes your search strategy more valid and will be useful if the search needs to be carried out again at a later date. Discussion of the 'hits' obtained and the selection process used to identify articles for closer study will also provide an audit trail. Having an audit trail is important if someone wants to repeat your review. Below is one way you could write up the databases you have searched.

- Cumulative Index to Nursing and Allied Health Literature (CINAHL) (1982 to 12/2015)
- MEDLINE (1996 to 12/2015)
- British Nursing Index (BNI) (1994 to 12/2015)
- Allied and Complementary Medicine Database (AMED) (1986 to 12/2015)
- Proquest (1990 to 12/2015)
- PsycINFO (2000 to 12/2015)
- Scopus (1990 to 12/2015)
- EMBASE (1988 to 12/2015)
- Science Direct (1990 to 12/2015)
- PubMed (1996 to 12/2015)
- Internurse (1996 to 12/2015)
- Health Management Information Consortium (HMIC) (12/2015)

Practice session 6.4

Try to document the search strategy for your own research question, using the format in Box 6.9.

Box 6.9   Template to use for documenting your search strategy

Database	Dates covered	Date searched	Hits	Full record/titles and abstracts	Notes

🔑 Key points

- The aim of a comprehensive and systematic search is to generate a comprehensive list of primary studies, both published and unpublished, which may be suitable for answering the proposed research question.

- Try to retrieve all studies (or as many as possible) pertaining to the specific question that your review is addressing, searching as widely as possible from a whole range of sources.

- It is necessary to search a wide variety of databases and internet search engines as well as hand searching and grey literature.

- Problems with searching include publication bias and language.

- Publication bias means that positive results tend to be published more frequently than negative results in journals.

- Language bias refers to the fact that positive results are more likely to be published in English.

- Bias may also relate to the geographical coverage of journals and databases.

- Key activities include reading reference lists, hand searching, accessing grey literature and getting in touch with authors of key articles.

- There are six steps involved in converting the review question into a comprehensive search strategy.

- Step 1 is to write out the research question and identify the PICO (population, intervention, comparative intervention, outcomes) or PEO (population, exposure, outcomes) component parts.

- Step 2 is to identify any synonyms (words that mean the same thing) for all the component parts (P, I, C, O or P, E, O) of the review question.

- Step 3 is to identify truncations and abbreviations.

- Step 4 is to develop a search strategy string (list of words) to input into the different databases.

- Step 6 is to undertake your comprehensive search using all sources of information.

- Step 6 is to save your searches.

Summary

This chapter discussed the importance, the rationale and the aims of undertaking a comprehensive and systematic search. The chapter described the key factors to be considered when undertaking a comprehensive search. The six steps involved in converting your review question into a comprehensive search strategy were described in detail.

Question and Answer (Q&A)

(Q) Is there any support available to help me with searching for the evidence?

(A) There are useful and inexpensive ways available to help support you with searching the evidence.

- Seeing if there are any literature searching sessions available at your local hospital and or university library.
- Making contact with the librarian for a one to one tutorial.
- You could make contact with someone who has undertaken a systematic review within your place of work.

7

Working with your primary papers: Stage 1 – Selecting the studies to include in your systematic review

Overview

- Methods of the review
- Selecting the appropriate papers to answer your review question
- Templates to select the papers for your own systematic literature review

Methods of the review

The methods of the review comprises three separate stages detailed in Box 7.1. These are further detailed in Figure 7.1. This chapter details Stage 1, where there are two steps to doing this: Step 1 is based on selecting the papers based on the titles and abstracts only and Step 2 involves selecting the papers based on reading the full paper (Figure 7.2).

Selecting the appropriate papers to answer your review question

Once you have conducted your search and specified your inclusion and exclusion criteria, the next step in conducting a systematic literature review is to select the studies that meet all your predetermined selection criteria. The actual process of how you select the studies to include in your review needs to be described in sufficient methodological detail to enable the steps to be replicated and thus ensure the whole process

---

Box 7.1 Methods of the review

When describing the methods of your review you will need to give details of the following **three separate stages**.

Stage 1: Describe how the process of selecting the papers for inclusion in your review will be carried out. This stage has two steps.

Stage 2: Describe how the process for the assessment of methodological quality of your papers will be carried out.

Stage 3: Describe how the process of extracting data from your papers will be carried out.

Stage 1	Selecting your papers	Step 1	Step 2
		(Based on titles & abstracts)	(Based on reading full papers)
Stage 2	Appraising your papers using a specific framework such as Caldwell et al., Critical Appraisal Skills Programme (CASP), McMasters		
Stage 3	Extracting data from your paper		

Figure 7.1 The three stages and steps of working with your primary papers.

Before you start
A standardized form needs to be made for ALL steps
This is important to standardize assessments between one paper and another
(i.e. improves inter- and intra-rater reliability)

Stage 1 – Step 1

At this point you have a large collection of abstracts, articles and papers from your search
1st Step – this selection is based on titles and abstracts ONLY considering the criteria of:

- type of study
- participants
- intervention
- comparative group
- outcome measures

using the standardized inclusion criteria FORM. Remember PICOS!
First selection can result in exclusion, inclusion or no decision on the title and abstract

Stage 1 – Step 2

This step is the same as for Step 1 but using the full papers. Second selection can result only in inclusion or exclusion of the full papers.

Figure 7.2 Flow diagram depicting the selection process.

is transparent. This will enable the appropriateness of the methods used to be easily evaluated and duplicated. This part of the review aims to filter out any irrelevant articles (Torgerson 2003).

The process of selecting studies for inclusion or exclusion in the review consists of two phases; the first phase involves sifting through the titles and abstracts of all the articles retrieved from the search, screening them systematically and selecting those that meet the predetermined inclusion criteria.

The second phase involves reading the full text of each identified article. For both phases it is useful to make an appropriate *research paper selection form* to help you standardize the way you select the articles that meet your predetermined criteria. This helps to make sure that you are always selecting the papers in the same way (i.e. it standardizes the process) and it also helps to improve the validity or truthfulness of the results.

Practical Tip

Developing a good study selection review template from the outset will enhance the quality and outcome of the review and make the process much simpler.

To explain how you make the paper selection form, let's look at examples from the three case studies used throughout this book on domestic violence (Mary), scoliosis (Cheryl) and witnessed resuscitation (Sue). Chapter 5 described how to specify your inclusion and exclusion criteria. In essence, to make your paper selection form all you need to do is copy the inclusion criteria and then turn these criteria into questions.

Ⓜ In the example of Mary's review, Mary starts by finding the electronic copy of her inclusion and exclusion criteria and copies the first two columns – the column entitled PICO components and the inclusion criteria column. Mary then turns all her original listed inclusion criteria statements into questions (usually this can be as simple as adding a question mark) as can be seen in Tables 7.1 and 7.2.

Mary has added another row to the bottom of her table to record the action with the rationale she will take and she has also added another column to the right side of the table (the decision column) to enable her to write whether or not that specific title and abstract meet the criteria (see Table 7.2) Mary's answers can be only one out of a possible three: yes, the paper meets these criteria and is denoted by (Y), no, the paper does not meet these criteria and is denoted by (N), or undecided as to whether this paper meets the inclusion criteria or not and is denoted by (U). If Mary is undecided, she will need to read the whole paper as well as ask a colleague or a supervisor for their opinion.

Practical Tip

It is important to test your paper selection form on a couple of articles to make sure that it is fit for purpose (this is similar to conducting a pilot study when doing primary research).

Ⓜ **Table 7.1** An example of Mary's inclusion and exclusion criteria

PICO components	Inclusion criteria	Exclusion criteria
Population	Women Adults >18 Experiencing or have experienced domestic violence in the past	Men, children and teenagers Women in lesbian relationships Women with disabilities Pregnant women
Intervention	Advocacy (conducted within or outside of health setting) Community programmes (need to include a clear definition of these)	Not formal cognitive–behavioural therapy
Comparative intervention	Usual (GP) treatment (usually this means no treatment for domestic violence)	Other interventions Alternative therapies
Outcomes Quantitative	Validated quality of life scales (need to specify which ones)	Experiences only on domestic violence or on children only

Ⓜ **Table 7.2** An example of how Mary could write her study selection form

Paper number:	Title	Authors
PICO components	Inclusion criteria	Decision: Yes, No, Undecided
Population	Women? Adults >18? Experiencing or have experienced domestic violence in the past?	
Intervention	Advocacy (conducted within or outside of health setting)? Community programmes?	
Comparative intervention	Usual (GP) treatment (usually this means no treatment for domestic violence)?	
Outcomes	Quality of life?	
Action (with rationale)	Include (read full article) Exclude or Undecided	

Although it is perfectly possible to select your papers on your own, it is important to remember that it would strengthen the validity (truthfulness) of your results if you can ask a friend or colleague to select the papers independently to see if they obtain the same results (Torgerson 2003; Petticrew and Roberts 2006). If you cannot find anyone, you should just acknowledge this.

§ Sue decided to use a slightly different format for her form (Table 7.3). She has decided she wants to use one form to select a number of studies. Although she will use less paper, this format does have a few limitations. She will be restricted in the amount of detail that she can include on her form and she will need to add a key to the bottom of the form, to clarify which specific paper each number on the top row of the form represents. It may also be difficult for her to write any specific queries that may arise from assessing each of her criteria for all her papers.

§ **Table 7.3** Example of Sue's first selection of papers based on title and abstract only

Paper and abstract number:	1	2	3	4	5	6	7	8	9	10	11	12
Population												
Adult patients	Y	N	?									
Age >18												
OR												
Family members OR	Y	Y	Y									
Healthcare professionals	Y	Y	Y									
Exposure												
Witnessed cardiopulmonary resuscitation or invasive procedures	Y	Y	?									
Outcomes												
Patient's experience of exposure	Y	Y	Y									
Family members' experience of exposure	Y	Y	Y									
Healthcare professionals' experience of exposure	Y	Y	Y									
Type of study												
Qualitative research	Y	N	Y									
*Action	Y	N	U									

*Action – Rationale: Y – Yes: fits criteria; N – No: does not fit criteria; U – Unsure: read paper.

After Sue has looked at three titles and abstracts, she fills in the first three columns on her selection form that represent these three papers (Table 7.3). In column 1 all the criteria have been met and Sue's overall decision (the action at the bottom) is to include the paper. In column 2 the action is to exclude the paper as two of the criteria have not been met. In column 3 there are two question marks, which means that Sue is undecided and needs to read the full paper and repeat the process. If she is still undecided after reading the full paper, she will need to consult with a colleague or supervisor. In summary the first phase can result in including an article, rejecting it or being undecided (Higgins and Deeks 2009).

Once Sue has finished the first part of the selection process, she will have a pile of abstracts that she has definitely decided to include, another pile about which she is uncertain and a third pile of abstracts that she has rejected. The first two piles must now be examined more closely for the second phase. This means obtaining full copies of the papers, reading them and making a decision regarding whether they meet the inclusion criteria that have been pre-set (Higgins and Deeks 2009).

Ⓒ Cheryl's paper selection form for review of adolescent patients with idiopathic scoliosis is shown in Table 7.4.

Ⓒ **Table 7.4** Cheryl's example for writing down the selection criteria for her review

Bibliographic details of paper	Inclusion	Decision: Yes, No, Undecided
Clinical population/ diagnosis	Patients with adolescent idiopathic scoliosis?	
Age	Ages 10–18? Or until the end of bone growth? Measured by an x-ray of the wrist or pelvis?	
Intervention	Rigid brace? Semi-rigid brace? Elastic brace? Worn for how many hours per day? How many days per week? How many years?	
Comparative intervention	Exercise? Rigid brace? Semi-rigid brace? Soft brace? Electrical stimulation? Surgery?	
Outcomes	Progression of scoliosis as measured by: • Cobb angle in degrees? • Number of patients who have progressed by more than five degrees Cobb? Quality of life and disability as measured by? Specific validated quality of life questionnaires such as: • SRS-22 (Asher et al. 2003)? • SF-36 (Lai et al. 2006)? • BSSK (Weiss et al. 2006)? Back pain as measured by: • Validated visual analogue scales? • Use of medication? • Adverse effects?	

Templates to select the papers for your own systematic literature review

---

Practice session 7.1

You have probably saved a number of papers from your searches and printed them out. Based on your own review question, select the appropriate template for either the PICO (Box 7.2) or PEO (Box 7.3) format to decide which of your primary research papers should be included, which should be excluded and which ones you are still undecided about. Once you have done this, you can go on to the next part of the study and appraise the methodological quality of your papers.

Box 7.2   PICO template to use for your own selection of papers

Bibliographic details of paper *(Fill in the details of the paper you are evaluating here)*

	Inclusion criteria	*Yes*	*No*	*Undecided*
Participants	*(This is where you write down the criteria for your population details, diagnosis, age etc.)*			
Intervention	*(Here you write down the specific criteria for your intervention)*			
Comparative intervention	*(Same but for comparative group)*			

(continued)

Box 7.2   Continued

	Inclusion criteria	Yes	No	Undecided
Outcomes	(Write down the specific outcomes you are looking for)			
Type of study	Write down the specific research designs you will be including			
Action (with rationale)	The action will be yes, no or undecided for the first phase and yes or no only for the second phase			

Box 7.3   PEO template to use for your own selection of papers

Bibliographic details of paper

Abstract number	1	2	3	4	5	6	7
Population							
Exposure							
Outcomes							
Type of studies							
*Action							

*Action – Rationale: Y – Yes: fits criteria; N – No: does not fit criteria; U – Undecided, read full paper

Key points

- The first phase involves sifting through the titles and abstracts of all the articles retrieved from the search, screening them systematically and selecting those that meet the predetermined inclusion criteria.

- For this phase it is useful to make an appropriate research paper selection form to help you standardize the way you select the articles.

Summary

This chapter focused on the first of three main stages that are involved in working with your primary research papers. The first stage includes ways of selecting appropriate papers to answer your review question. This step is conducted in two parts: select your papers based on the title and abstract according to your predetermined criteria, then repeat this process when reading the full paper. Developing and using the templates detailed in the chapter will enhance this aspect of the review.

Question and Answer (Q&A)

(Q) Are there any useful resources to aid the review process?

(A) There are several useful resources available to aid you in undertaking a quality review of the articles. For example the Joanna Briggs Institute and York Centre for Reviews and Dissemination both offer online resources and manuals highlighting the review process.

8

Working with your primary papers: Stage 2 – Appraising the methodological quality of your included research studies

Overview

- Appraising the methodological quality of the research papers that you have selected
- Worked example using the Caldwell et al. framework to critique a nursing paper

Appraising the methodological quality of the research papers that you have selected

As we explained in the previous chapter, the methods of review section of your review should cover the three separate stages detailed in Box 8.1. This chapter details Stage 2, focusing on how to identify and critique methodological quality.

Box 8.1   Methods of the review

In this section you need to give details of the following three separate stages.

Stage 1: The process of selecting the papers for inclusion in the systematic review. This stage has two steps.

Stage 2: The process for the assessment of methodological quality will be carried out.

Stage 3: The process for the proposed data extraction strategy.

Appraising 'study quality' is often used interchangeably with assessing the 'internal validity', which is the extent to which a study is free from methodological biases (Petticrew and Roberts 2006) or the degree to which the results of a study are likely to approximate the 'truth' (Higgins and Deeks 2009). In the context of systematic reviews, quality refers to the methodological quality – the internal and external validity of quantitative studies. Jadad (1998) suggested that the following points may be relevant when assessing the quality of RCTs.

- Relevance of the research question.
- Internal validity of the trial – the degree to which the trial design, conduct, analysis and presentation have minimized or avoided bias.
- External validity – the extent to which findings are generalizable.
- Appropriateness of the data analysis and presentation.
- Ethical implications of the intervention the paper evaluated. This refers to the ethics in the included papers within the review, for example was informed consent obtained?

The criteria for qualitative articles are different. Qualitative articles are often judged with regard to authenticity and trustworthiness, rather than validity or reliability (please see Figure 8.1 and guidelines below for a more detailed explanation). Table 8.1 shows the common features of research critique frameworks for both quantitative and qualitative studies.

Appraising the quality of articles is crucial as it allows the exploration of how differences in quality might explain differences in the study results, and it will also guide the interpretation of the findings and their value to practice. There are a number of practical issues to consider when appraising a study (Centre for Reviews and Dissemination 2008). These include stating who will be assessing the quality of the studies, how many reviewers will be involved, what checklist or scale will be used for quality assessment and how the reviewers will resolve disagreements. Involvement of a colleague or a supervisor is important (if possible) to ensure that all articles are appropriately critiqued.

The quality of evidence and conclusions generated by a systematic literature review for nursing practice depends entirely on the quality of the primary studies that

Table 8.1 Common features of research critique frameworks

Quantitative	Qualitative
Research design	Philosophical background
Experimental hypothesis	Research design
Operational definitions	Concepts
Population	Context
Sample	Sample
Sampling	Sampling
Validity/reliability of data collection	Auditability of data collection
Data analysis	Credibility/confirmability of data analysis
Generalizability	Transferability

Source: Reprinted from Caldwell, K., Henshaw, L. and Taylor, G. (2011) Developing a framework for critiquing health research: an early evaluation. *Nurse Education Today* 31 (8): e1–7, with permission from Elsevier.

make up the review. This quality assessment is one of the key features that sets apart a systematic review from a narrative review. To assess the quality of primary articles, a number of assessment tools are available that are easily accessible online (Box 8.2). It is important to use appropriate checklists or scales for the type of study design to be evaluated. Box 8.2 lists some of the scales that can be used to evaluate randomized and non-randomized studies, as well as websites where critical appraisal forms for different study designs can be found. There is a large range of critical appraisal tools available in the literature.

Box 8.2   Websites for some common appraisal frameworks

- Critical Appraisal Skills Programme:
  http://www.casp-uk.net/
- McMaster University Evidence-Based Practice Research Group:
  http://srs-mcmaster.ca/research/evidence-based-practice-research-group
- Newcastle-Ottawa Scale (NOS) for assessing the quality of non-randomized studies in meta-analysis:
  http://www.ohri.ca/programs/clinical_epidemiology/oxford.asp

---

Practical Tip

Using recognized checklists, scales and/or critical appraisal tools can save you lots of time in undertaking your review. Essentially you are not developing these from scratch.

Worked examples of both quantitative and qualitative critiques can be found in Chapters 4–6 of *The Evidence-Based Practice Manual for Nurses* (Craig and Smyth 2007). One set of critical appraisal forms that we often recommend to students is the McMaster framework for critiquing qualitative or quantitative studies (see Box 8.2). This framework includes excellent guidelines on how to conduct the different kinds of critical appraisals for both quantitative and qualitative research and provides advice for answering each of the questions. Although devised by occupational therapists, the framework is written in basic terms that can be understood by any clinician, researcher and student.

Another framework developed by Caldwell et al. (2011) for nursing students has combined both quantitative and qualitative appraisal questions into one form that can be used for any type of research design. The framework comes with some guidelines that give an explanation of each item. Nursing students have found this framework (Figure 8.1) together with the guidelines (some of which are given here) both easy to use and to follow. The critical appraisal questions that follow are from Caldwell et al. (2011).

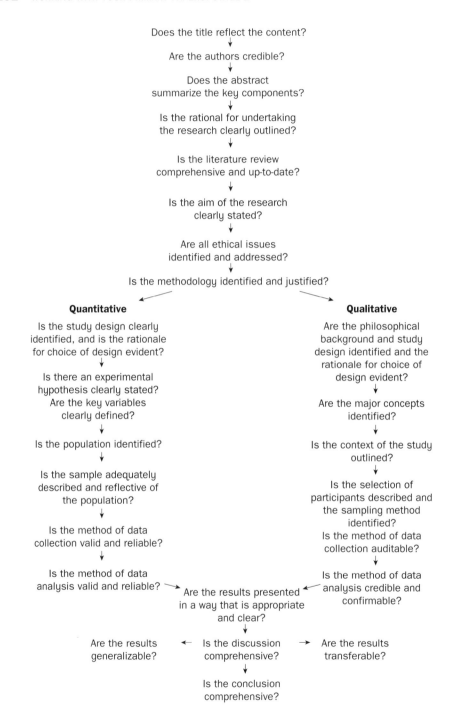

Figure 8.1 Framework by Caldwell et al. (2011).

Source: Reprinted from Caldwell, K., Henshaw, L. and Taylor, G. (2011) Developing a framework for critiquing health research: an early evaluation. *Nurse Education Today* 31 (8): e1–7, with permission from Elsevier.

- **Does the title reflect the content?** The title should be informative and indicate the focus of the study. It should allow the reader to easily interpret the content of the study. An inaccurate or misleading title can confuse the reader.

- **Are the authors credible?** Researchers should hold appropriate academic qualifications and be linked to a professional field relevant to the research.

- **Does the abstract summarize the key components?** The abstract should provide a short summary of the study. It should include the aim of the study, outline of the methodology and the main findings. The purpose of the abstract is to allow the reader to decide if the study is of interest to them.

- **Is the rationale for undertaking the research clearly outlined?** The author should present a clear rationale for the research, setting it in context of any current issues and knowledge of the topic to date.

- **Is the literature review comprehensive and up-to-date?** The literature review should reflect the current state of knowledge relevant to the study and identify any gaps or conflicts. It should include key or classic studies on the topic as well as up-to-date literature. There should be a balance of primary and secondary sources.

- **Is the aim of the research clearly stated?** The aim of the study should be clearly stated and should convey what the researcher is setting out to achieve.

- **Are all ethical issues identified and addressed?** Ethical issues pertinent to the study should be discussed. The researcher should identify how the rights of informants have been protected and informed consent obtained. If the research is conducted within the National Health Service (NHS), there should be indication of local research ethics committee approval.

- **Is the methodology identified and justified?** The researcher should make clear which research strategy they are adopting, i.e. qualitative or quantitative. A clear rationale for the choice should also be provided, so that the reader can judge whether the chosen strategy is appropriate for the study. At this point the student is asked to look specifically at the questions that apply to the paradigm appropriate to the study they are critiquing.

- **Are the results presented in a way that is appropriate and clear?** Presentation of data should be clear, easily interpreted and consistent.

- **Is the discussion comprehensive?** In quantitative studies the results and discussion are presented separately. In qualitative studies these may be integrated. Whatever the mode of presentation, the researcher should compare and contrast the findings with that of previous research on the topic. The discussion should be balanced and avoid subjectivity.

- **Is the conclusion comprehensive?** Conclusions must be supported by the findings. The researcher should identify any limitations to the study. There may also be recommendations for further research or, if appropriate, implications for practice in the relevant field.

To complete your critique, the final questions that you need to address are applied to both quantitative and qualitative studies (see Table 8.2).

Table 8.2 Questions specifically relevant to either quantitative or qualitative research

Quantitative	Qualitative
Is the design clearly identified and a rationale provided? The design of the study, e.g. survey experiment, should be identified and justified. As with the choice of strategy, the reader needs to consider whether the design is appropriate for the research undertaken.	*Are the philosophical background and study design identified and the rationale for choice evident?* The design of the study, e.g. phenomenology, ethnography, should be identified and the philosophical background and rationale discussed. The reader needs to consider if it is appropriate to meet the aims of the study.
Is there an experimental hypothesis clearly stated and are the key variables identified? In experimental research, the researcher should provide a hypothesis. This should clearly identify the independent and dependent variables, and state their relationship and the intent of the study. In survey research the researcher may choose to provide a hypothesis, but it is not essential, and alternatively a research question or aim may be provided.	*Are the major concepts identified?* The researchers should make clear what the major concepts are, but they might not define them. The purpose of the study is to explore the concepts from the perspective of the participants.
Is the population identified? The population is the total number of units from which the researcher can gather data. It may be individuals, organizations or documentation. Whatever the unit, it must be clearly identified.	*Is the context of the study outlined?* The researcher should provide a description of the context of the study, how the study sites were determined and how the participants were selected.
Is the sample adequately described and reflective of the population? Both the method of sampling and the size of the sample should be stated so that the reader can judge whether the sample is representative of the population and sufficiently large to eliminate bias.	*Is the selection of the participants described and sampling method identified?* Informants are selected for their relevant knowledge or experience. Representativeness is not a criteria and purposive sampling is often used. Sample size may be determined through saturation.
Is the method of data collection valid and reliable? The process of data collection should be described. The tools or instruments must be appropriate to the aims of the study and the researcher should identify how reliability and validity were assured.	*Is the method of data collection auditable?* Data collection methods should be described, and be appropriate to the aims of the study. The researcher should describe how they assured that the method is auditable.
Is the method of data analysis valid and reliable? The method of data analysis must be described and justified. Any statistical test used should be appropriate for the data involved.	*Is the method of data analysis credible and confirmable?* The data analysis strategy should be identified; what processes were used to identify patterns and themes? The researcher should identify how credibility and confirmability have been addressed.

Source: Reprinted from Caldwell, K., Henshaw, L. and Taylor, G. (2011) Developing a framework for critiquing health research: an early evaluation. *Nurse Education Today* 31 (8): e1–7, with permission from Elsevier.

The questions posed in Figure 8.1 that are specifically relevant to either quantitative or qualitative research are discussed further below. We have included a worked example using the Caldwell et al. (2011) framework.

Worked example using the Caldwell et al. framework to critique a nursing paper

By now you should have familiarized yourself with and learnt the questions to ask when critiquing both quantitative and/or qualitative papers. Below you will find a worked example of a critique of a research paper taken from the nursing literature. We hope that this will provide a useful illustration of how to critique a paper. We also feel this may help you to think through the issues that need to be considered to comprehensively critique a paper appropriately.

The name of the paper is: Biofeedback Intervention for Stress and Anxiety among Nursing Students: A Randomized Controlled Trial (http://www.ncbi.nlm.nih.gov/pmc/articles/PMC3395228/). This paper was written by P. Ratanasiripong, N. Ratanasiripong and D. Kathalae. It is published in the International Scholarly Research Network (ISRN) Nursing Volume 2012, Article ID 827972 and is 5 pages long. (It is very easy to locate the full text of this paper just by typing the title into Google.) See Table 8.3 for the critique.

Action during and following the completion of your critique

An 'important' point to remember is the fact that you should score the various questions while you are doing your critique. Once you have completed the critique you need to provide a holistic assessment of whether the quality of this paper was Excellent, High, Medium, Low or Very Low. The lowest score is 1 and the highest 3 for each individual question. You then need to total the scores for each question providing a total score for the paper. For this paper a score of 26/36 was achieved indicating the quality of the paper could have been improved – in other words, there were many errors. In research terms this could be stated as a significant amount of bias found within the study. (Please refer to Chapter 10 for further discussion).

Practice session 8.1

Once you have read through the framework and guidelines (Caldwell et al. 2011), work through the appropriate questions for your type of paper (qualitative or quantitative) and try to critique them. Alternatively, you can select either the quantitative or the qualitative critical appraisal forms available on the McMaster site and work through those using their guidelines. Visit their site at: http://srs-mcmaster.ca/research/evidence-based-practice-research-group.

Table 8.3 Worked example of a critique using the Caldwell et al. framework questions for the paper 'Biofeedback Intervention for Stress and Anxiety among Nursing Students: A Randomized Controlled Trial'

	Caldwell Framework questions	Evaluation	Score
1	Does the title reflect the content?	Yes, the title of this paper is reflective of the content of the paper. The PICO components are clearly stated as well as the research design of the study which is a randomized controlled trial (RCT). Although the comparative intervention is not included in the title it is clear that there must be a comparative intervention as the research design is an RCT. However, it is unclear from the title what the comparative intervention is. It is also unclear from the title what specific biofeedback machine was used.	1
2	Are the authors credible?	Although the professional titles as well as the qualifications of the authors cannot be found on the paper, the fact that all three authors' addresses are universities suggests that they are lecturers or assistant professors with appropriate qualifications. It would have been helpful, however, for the editor/s of the journal to have included the qualifications of the authors to enable readers to better appraise the authors' credibility.	1
3	Does the abstract summarize the key components?	Yes, the abstract provided for this paper includes a structured abstract with sub-headings so the purpose, methods, results and conclusions are very clear. It is unclear from the abstract, however, what the specific biofeedback device is.	1
4	Is the rational, for undertaking the research clearly outlined?	Yes, this was clearly explained by describing what previous studies had and had not been investigated (i.e. the gap in the literature was clearly highlighted. The authors stated that no recent studies had been conducted with the new generation of portable biofeedback equipment that addressed nursing students' stress and anxiety, however, the reader is left to take this statement at face value without being clear as to how comprehensive and how in-depth the search for papers was.	2
5	Is the literature review comprehensive and up to date?	The authors have thoroughly described previous studies in the area and the papers appear to be up to date.	2
6	Is the aim of the study clearly stated?	The purpose is clearly described in the abstract, however, I could not find it restated within the main paper after the background section	2

	Caldwell Framework questions	Evaluation	Score
7	Are all ethical issues identified and addressed?	Yes, all ethical issues appear to have been identified and addressed. The study was approved by the nursing colleges institutional review board for ethical approval and all participants in the study volunteered to take part and signed the informed consent forms.	2
8	Is the methodology identified and addressed?	Yes, the methodology was very clearly identified and addressed.	1
9	Is the design clearly identified and a rationale provided?	Yes, the research design was appropriately identified as an RCT but a rationale was not provided.	1
10	Is there an experimental hypothesis clearly stated and are the key variables identified?	No, the experimental hypothesis was not specifically stated but the purpose of the study was very clearly stated. However, as stated in the left column of Table 8.2 it is not essential to do this for surveys. The key variables were not explicitly stated, however, both the independent variable (the biofeedback intervention) as well as the dependent variables (stress and anxiety) were described in depth.	1
11	Is the population identified?	Yes, the population was clearly identified. They consisted of 60 second-year baccalaureate nursing students aged between 18 and 21 years old.	2
12	Is the sample adequately described and reflective of the population?	Yes, both the method of sampling and the size of the sample were clearly described so the reader could judge that the sample was representative of the population and sufficiently large to eliminate bias. In fact the authors also calculated an *a priori* power analysis that identified at least 60 participants were needed.	2
13	Is the method of data collection valid and reliable?	Yes, the method of data collection appeared to be valid and reliable with some exceptions; it was unclear precisely how the participants were randomly allocated to the biofeedback or the comparison intervention (i.e. nothing). This could have led to allocation bias. Additionally the instrument should have been clearly described in a separate instrumentation section that needed to be located before the procedure section. The internal consistency of both the anxiety and stress scales were discussed. It is unclear, however, whether the reliability of the biofeedback device was assessed.	1

	Caldwell Framework questions	Evaluation	Score
14	Is the method of data analysis valid and reliable? The method of data analysis must be described and justified. Any statistical test used should be appropriate for the data involved.	The method of data analysis was described and justified. However, more appropriate tests could have been selected to enhance the validity of the study. The statistical tests used were adequate for the data involved but involved conducting more tests than necessary, which could have led to a type 1 error (this is where the results indicate that the intervention is effective when in reality it is not). For example, a more appropriate test that would have assessed all the differences between the four areas below could have been applied: 1. Pre-intervention biofeedback and comparative group 2. Post-intervention biofeedback and comparison group 3. Differences between the pre- and post-biofeedback data, and 4. Differences between the pre- and post-comparative intervention data In this instance the most appropriate statistical test for this (assuming the data was normally distributed) would have been a 2 way ANOVA with repeated measures and a *post hoc* test. A statistically significant ANOVA test lets you know that there are significant differences between different groups but it does not let you know specifically which groups are significantly different, so that is why you need a *post hoc* test. Usually this is either the Bonferroni test or the Tukey *post hoc* test.	1
15	Are the results presented in a way that is appropriate and clear?	Yes the results were presented very clearly by the use of graphs and tables that were clearly labelled and explained within the text. A good use of colour was made to differentiate between the biofeedback and the comparison groups.	2
16	Is the discussion comprehensive?	Partly.	1
17	Is the conclusion comprehensive?	Yes, the conclusions were comprehensive. The limitations of the study were clearly discussed as were the implications for nursing practice. Recommendations were appropriately made for further research in this field.	2
18	Are the results generalizable?	Yes and no. Yes the results are definitely generalizable to other nursing schools within Thailand, however, we do not know if they are generalizable to other nursing schools in different countries as these were not included within this study although the assumption is that they would be.	1

26/36

🔑 Key points

- A quality assessment of your primary papers is one of the key features that sets apart a systematic review from a narrative review.

- To assess the quality of primary articles, a number of assessment tools are available that are easily accessible online or you can use the one included in this chapter.

- It is important to use appropriate checklists or scales for the type of study design to be evaluated.

Summary

This chapter discussed the second main stage involved in working with your primary research papers. Stage 2 detailed the importance of appraising the methodological quality of your articles and included useful tools and frameworks to aid you in the process. The importance of using a form or framework to standardize and increase the reliability and validity for all stages of the process is clarified by using relevant examples from nursing practice.

Question and Answer (Q&A)

(Q) Is there any one critical appraisal framework available that I should use to review the literature?

(A) There are numerous critical appraisal frameworks available for use to aid you with your review of the articles. Prior to undertaking the review we would suggest that you look at some of the various frameworks and find one which suits you best. The only way to establish which one is best for you is to review and complete these before you commence your systematic review. The Caldwell et al. (2011) framework discussed above can be used to appraise both quantitative and qualitative research, whereas the McMaster's framework is useful because this framework also provides guidelines to help you fill in the form in the event that you may need to remind yourself of basic research concepts.

9

Working with your primary papers: Stage 3 – Extracting the data from your included papers

Overview

- Extracting the appropriate data from your research papers
- The process for Mary's quantitative systematic literature review on domestic violence
- The process for Sue's qualitative systematic literature review on witnessed resuscitation

Extracting the appropriate data from your research papers

The methods section of your review needs to cover the three stages detailed in Box 9.1. This chapter details Stage 3, focusing on how to extract the right data from the papers you have selected.

Box 9.1 Methods of the review

In this section you need to give details of the following **three separate stages**.

Stage 1: The process of selecting the papers for inclusion in the systematic review. This stage has two steps

Stage 2: The process for the assessment of methodological quality will be carried out.

Stage 3: The process for the proposed data extraction strategy.

The data extraction phase is perhaps the most challenging aspect of the methodology. Data extraction involves going back to the primary articles and highlighting the relevant information that will answer the research question. Normally, this involves extracting data related to the population included, the intervention, comparative intervention and particularly the outcomes (the PICO components). To standardize this process and improve the validity of the results, it is crucial to compile a data extraction form. As with the selection form previously described, it is important to pilot the form on one or two of the articles to ensure it is useful and appropriate (Higgins and Deeks 2009). An example of the forms and how these can be applied in practice are demonstrated in both Mary and Sue's case studies.

The process for Mary's quantitative systematic literature review on domestic violence

Ⓜ Let us first consider Mary's quantitative case study example on domestic violence. Mary needs to look back at the PICO form she made when selecting her articles, presented earlier in Chapter 7. She knows that all the articles included in the final selection are relevant to the research question and have met the inclusion criteria. In the data extraction form, it is important that she extracts all the relevant information to enable her to answer her question related to women's quality of life. As well as collecting information on the population, intervention and control group, Mary will need to collect information on the outcomes. Table 9.1 provides an example of what one of Mary's data extraction forms might look like, together with our comments on what Mary needs to do in each section.

Ⓜ **Table 9.1** Example of Mary's data extraction form

Date of data extraction: 23/4/11 *(here Mary writes down the date when she fills in the form)*
Reviewer: Mary Smith *(here she writes her name as the reviewer of the paper)*
Bibliographic details of study: *(here she writes the reference for the paper)*
Jones, J. (2008) The effect of advocacy interventions compared to usual care on abused women's quality of life. *Journal of Clinical Nursing* 10 (5): 345–352.
Purpose of study: *(here she writes down the purpose of the paper from which she is extracting the data)*
The purpose of the study is to evaluate the effectiveness of a community advocacy programme as compared with usual care on abused women's quality of life.
Study design: *(here she writes down the study design – usually this can be found in the abstract)*
Randomized controlled trial
Population (sample): *(here she summarizes the information about the sample used in the paper)*
60 women who were experiencing or had previously experienced domestic violence were included in the study. The women were randomly allocated to either the intervention group (*n*=30) or the control group who received usual care (*n*=30).
Intervention: *(Mary summarizes what the intervention was)*
Women attended an advocacy group once a week over 12 weeks. Group meetings provided support and help for women on all aspects relevant to domestic violence.
Comparative intervention: *(the same for the comparative intervention)*
The women in this group received usual care.
Outcomes: *(This part is very important. Mary needs to search for the results of the study in the results section of the article. As her outcomes relate to quality of life scales she needs to copy the pre- and post-intervention values for both the advocacy group and the usual care group as seen below. In this case the results of this paper have been extracted.)*
    SF-36 quality of life scales
    Pre-intervention advocacy group 30/50 (50 is the average rate for healthy individuals)
    Post-intervention advocacy group 40/50
    Pre-intervention usual care group 29/50
    Post-intervention usual care group 30/50

The process for Sue's qualitative systematic literature review on witnessed resuscitation

§ Turning to Sue's qualitative literature review, Sue first needs to make a data extraction form. This part of the process is identical whether you are planning to extract qualitative or quantitative data. The key difference between the two types of data extraction forms (qualitative or quantitative) is that the outcomes section in a qualitative data extraction form will be inserted under the main themes that were decided upon for your review question when you were planning your protocol or plan and the data extracted will be the 'words or perceptions' of the population group(s) you have decided to include. For quantitative data extraction forms, it is numbers that are mostly extracted.

Sue has decided to include three different population groups as listed in Box 9.2. When constructing the outcomes section of her data extraction form, she also included a section where she would write down the page number, column number and line numbers of the words extracted (sentences and paragraphs that she will extract from her papers). This will let her know what part of the paper the excerpt came from and improve the audit trail of her review. Table 9.2 provides an example of what Sue's data extraction form looked like before she filled it in.

---

§ Box 9.2   Sue's proposed outcomes

- Outcome 1: Patient's experience of resuscitation and/or invasive procedures (Table 9.3)
- Outcome 2: Family members' experience of resuscitation and/or invasive procedures (Table 9.4)
- Outcome 3: Healthcare professionals' experience of resuscitation and/or invasive procedures (Table 9.5)

---

§ **Table 9.2** Sample data extraction form

Date of data extraction:	*(Today's date)*
Reviewer:	*(Your name)*
Bibliographical details of study:	*(Full reference of article including author, year and source)*
Purpose of study:	*(This is outlined by the author of the article)*
Study design:	*(Type of qualitative study utilized for purpose of the article)*
Population (sample):	*(This section outlines the description of the study sample characteristics as identified)*
Number Age – Ethnicity –	
Exposure:	*(Witnessed resuscitation and/or invasive procedures)*

§ **Table 9.3** Outcome 1: Patient's experience of resuscitation and/or invasive procedures

Page	Col.	Line	Data extracted	Subthemes

§ **Table 9.4** Outcome 2: Family members' experience of resuscitation and/or invasive procedures

Page	Col.	Line	Data extracted	Subthemes

§ **Table 9.5** Outcome 3: Healthcare professionals' experience of resuscitation and/or invasive procedures

Page	Col.	Line	Data extracted	Subthemes

Having completed the data extraction it is important to highlight and summarize the outcomes. The outcomes of Sue's case study are highlighted below.

Practical Tip

Our students found it really helped them to colour code all their different outcomes in different colours as this helped them to quickly know which outcome they were working with.

Once the data extraction form was ready, Sue was able to proceed with the data extraction process. There are a number of ways of extracting data from qualitative papers with no one way being dominant. The literature is somewhat controversial and vague within this area. Consequently, this has led to new researchers being unclear as to how precisely to proceed with extracting qualitative data.

Practical Tip

There are a number of qualitative frameworks currently available to aid with extracting qualitative data. Before starting your review it is important to look at those that are available and find one that you feel is appropriate for your review.

Below we have outlined one way of doing this but there are many different ways this can be done. The method described below has been adapted from Burnard's (1991) method of thematic analysis and follows the same methodology that you would use to analyse any qualitative data, for example interviews. Burnard (1991) has published an excellent detailed description of the steps involved in his article entitled 'A method of analysing interview transcripts in qualitative research'. In the next part of this chapter you will find a description for one process for extracting data from a research paper. It takes you through each step.

 ### Step 1

Before Sue starts extracting qualitative data (i.e. words and sentences) it is important that she reads the results section of her primary papers a number of times to become fully immersed in the data. The purpose of immersion is to become more fully aware of the 'lived world' of the participants and to try to see the world from the other person's perspective.

 ### Step 2

As part of her research question Sue has decided which specific themes she intends to look at as part of developing her review question. Sue is looking at the perspectives of three different population groups – the patients, the families and the healthcare professionals – and has colour coded them in three different colours. Sue's colour-coding scheme involves highlighting any perceptions in the primary research papers to do with patients in green, any families' perceptions in yellow and any healthcare professionals' perspectives in blue. This can be done either manually by using highlighter pens or electronically on the computer.

 ### Step 3

The next step is to cut out (either manually or electronically) all the text highlighted in different colours and paste it in the 'Data extracted' section of the form. In Sue's scenario, all green highlighted text related to patients will be inserted under Outcome 1 of the form, all yellow highlighted text related to family members will be inserted under Outcome 2 of the form and the same for Outcome 3. Eventually Sue will end up with all the data or text in the primary paper related to patients, family members and healthcare professionals under the appropriate headings and sections in the data extraction form (see Table 9.2). She also needs to make sure that she notes the page number, column number and line number from the primary paper as she will need this information when she refers to them in the results or discussion sections of her review. It is important to clarify your audit trail.

 ### Step 4

In the data extraction form, Sue writes down as many headings as necessary to describe all aspects of the content excluding 'dross'. Field and Morse (1985) state that the term 'dross' is used to denote any unusable fillers in an interview or paper, such as issues that are unrelated to the topic in hand. The headings or category system should account for almost all the category data. This phase is known as *open coding*, meaning that categories are generated freely (Burnard 1991: 462).

 ### Step 5

When Sue has written down all the categories for the results section, the next step is for her to look through the headings and to try to group them together under 'higher order' headings. Burnard (1991) explains that the aim here is to reduce the number of categories by 'collapsing' some of the ones that are similar into broader categories. For example, it could be decided that all the headings in the 'categories' column could be collapsed into one higher order heading as shown in Table 9.6.

§ **Table 9.6** Healthcare professionals' (HCPs') experience of resuscitation and/or invasive procedures

| | | | Outcome/theme 3 | | | |
| | | | Healthcare professionals' experience of resuscitation and/or invasive procedures | | | Higher order headings |
Page	Col.	Line	Data extracted	Open coding	Categories	
90	1	35–39	Other concerns stemmed from the insertion of chest drains, defibrillating, putting in tubes, inserting needles and intubation.	Concerns arising from insertion of diverse ⟶ medical devices	HCPs' concerns relating to ⟶ family's needs	HCPs' concerns for family needs and feelings during the procedure
91	1	1–3	All of these are invasive procedures ⟶ that are	Invasive procedures	Invasive and ⟶ abnormal procedures	
			'abnormal in their (the relatives') eyes, and therefore difficult for the relatives to witness.'	Abnormal procedures for relatives ⟶ / Difficult for families to witness	HCPs' concern for ⟶ families' feelings	

Step 6

The new list of categories are worked through and very similar headings are removed.

Step 7

This step is used to 'increase the validity of the categorizing method and to guard against researcher bias' (Burnard 1991: 493). It is important to ask one or two colleagues to independently generate the categories from the same research paper without looking at your own list. Once this has been done the categories are discussed and any changes made as necessary.

Step 8

When you have obtained a revised list, you need to reread the results section of the research paper and make sure that the final categories and subheadings still cover *all the relevant parts* of the results section. Then make any changes you think necessary.

Step 9

Once this has been done for one primary research paper, the same process is carried out for all the included papers. One of Sue's completed data extraction forms is shown in Table 9.7. The process of synthesizing the data extraction forms will be discussed in Chapter 10.

§ **Table 9.7** One of Sue's completed data extraction forms

Date of data extraction: 19 March 2011
Reviewer: SH
Bibliographical details of study: Goodenough, T. J. and Brysiewicz, P. (2003) 'Witnessed resuscitation: Exploring the attitudes and practices of the emergency staff working in Level I Emergency Departments in the province of KwaZulu-Natal'. *Curationis* 29 (2): 59–93 (supplied by the British Library)
Area: KwaZulu-Natal
Purpose of study: Explore the attitudes and practices of witnessed resuscitation by the staff working in Level I Emergency Departments in the province of KwaZulu-Natal
Study design: Qualitative survey
Setting: Emergency Department
Population:
Sample selection: Purposeful sample of six staff members from two different Level I Emergency Departments. From each of these hospitals the sample consisted of one medical officer, one registered nurse and one registered nurse in charge of the unit. All participants had to be employed in the department for more than six months in order to ensure they had experienced resuscitation procedures. This purposeful selection method was appropriate to the purpose and question as it identified a combination of attitudes from both clinical and managerial staff
Number: Six
Length of experience: Minimum 9 months to 8 years
Exposure: Resuscitation/invasive procedures
Outcome/theme 1: Healthcare professionals' experience of resuscitation and or invasive procedures

Page	Col.	Line	Data extracted	Subthemes
90 91	1 1	35–39 1–3	Other concerns stemmed from the insertion of chest drains, defibrillating, putting in tubes, inserting needles and intubation. All of these are invasive procedures that are 'abnormal in their (the relatives') eyes, and therefore difficult for the relatives to witness.'	Family needs Concern for families' feelings
90	2	29–31	The staff didn't think that the relatives should be present at the resuscitation of their loved one, and they said they would prefer not to be present at the resuscitation of their own family members. 'I totally disagree with allowing family members into the resuscitation room . . .' 'I don't think it's very nice.'	Family needs Concern for families' feelings

(Continued overleaf)

§ **Table 9.7** Continued

Outcome/theme 2: Patient's experience of resuscitation and/or invasive procedures				
Page	*Col.*	*Line*	*Data extracted*	*Subthemes*
92	1	1–10	When family members were present the patients felt loved, supported and less alone. One said, 'It would have been awful to be there alone and have no family there by your side. It would be even worse.'	Family presence
			Patients recounted that family members hugged and kissed them, held their hands, and listened to their fears.	Comfort measures
			One patient undergoing a lumbar puncture said: 'I was scared that it was going to hurt. I didn't want people going in my back. I was afraid. Having him there was so comforting.'	Reassurance from family members
91	1	22–28	Patients described themselves as being 'afraid, hurt, and in pain' during the emergency event. They related feeling safer and less scared when family members were there. 'The injuries were so severe . . . you can deal with a situation like that a lot better if you have the reinforcement of a loved one.' 'I was very scared. I thought I would never have a leg again. It was broken really badly. I thought I might die. I remember waking up and seeing all those doctors. I was like, Where am I? Something is wrong! I looked over and saw my dad and my mother. They were there to help me, to hold my hand, to give me a hug.'	Family presence Comfort measures Reassurance from parents' presence

Outcome/theme 3: Family members' experience of resuscitation and/or invasive procedures

Page	*Col.*	*Line*	*Data extracted*	*Subthemes*
59	2	20–21	'I couldn't not have been there, I needed to be with him and I was.' (Fran)	Family needs
59	2	23–28	'I felt useful during the event, I genuinely felt that I was contributing positively and that helps me a lot [pauses]. I can also recall that his eyes were looking at me, as though he knew it was me next to him . . . I was able to keep speaking to him – comforting him – I think!' (Jane)	Feeling conscious of presence Feeling useful during event
59	2	35–39	'John didn't know I was there, of course, he can't remember anything of the event for a good two weeks after . . . And, I didn't think at the time he would know that I was there. I just stood at the foot of his bed – so how could he possibly have known I was there?' (Ann)	Family needs Familiarity and support for patient

When Sue has extracted her data from one paper, she needs to repeat the process for all her included studies. Sue's data should now be synthesized, which means putting it all together or combining it. This is usually carried out by using tables or graphics for quantitative data or presenting them under themes for qualitative data. The ways of doing this will be discussed in Chapter 10.

𝔽 One of Fay's data extraction forms can be seen below in Figure 9.1.

CAUTI: Sterile Versus Non-sterile Catheter Insertion

DATA Extraction Form

Details of Study 8:

TITLE: Comparison of a Microbicidal Povidone-iodine gel and a placebo gel as catheter lubricants. (Author: Harrison, L H. (1980))
SOURCE: *The Journal of Urology,* 124 (3):pq 347–349.

Reviewer's Name: Fiona Bezzina   Date: 6th Sept 2008

Purpose of the study: to evaluate the Microbicidal effect and lubricating action of Povidone-iodine lubricating gel when used clinically as a catheter lubricant. Patient acceptance and tolerance, burning or stinging sensation, were also recorded.

Study Design: Cohort study

POPULATION:

Sample size: 50   (intervention group n=26; control group n=24)

Criteria of diagnosis (CAUTI or Bacteriuria): Urethral bacterial colony counts

Any Secondary diagnosis: Urinary Tract and/or Prostatic disorders

Inclusion/Exclusion Criteria: No information given on the inclusion criteria.
Exclusion criteria: Patients who were known to be sensitive to the ingredients of the test or the control gels; subjects who were on antibiotics and patients suffering from urethral burning, stinging or irritation or any medical problem requiring treatment that might have interfered with the results.

Type of Catheterisation: urethral, Intermittent and indwelling
Reason for catheterisation: Urinary tract or prostatic disorders
Setting: Nor clearly stated; probably in hospital.

INTERVENTION:

Experimental Intervention/s: Penis was held by an attendant and the glans was rinsed with sterile distilled water. Distal urethral swab was taken. Using sterile technique, povidone iodine gel was applied along the length of the catheter which was then inserted. Patient was asked about subjective sensation (burning or stinging sensation). 3 minutes post-insertion the catheter was withdrawn and another swab was taken from the portion of the catheter that previously was in contact with the urethra. All specimens were sent to the microbiology laboratory.
Duration of Intervention/s: 3 Minutes
Adverse Effects: None reported
Control Treatment/s: same protocol as experimental but K-Y jelly was used as lubricant.
Drop-outs: None reported

CAUTI: Sterile Versus Non-sterile Catheter Insertion

Study 8: Harrison (1980)   Data Extraction Form (Continued)

OUTCOMES:

CAUTI:

Number of UTI's (in Experimental and Control groups):

Bacteriuria (Urine sample):
Symptomatic UTI:
Combined Results:

> The pre-catheterisation geometric mean (the aver-
> age of the logarithim counts) was 9549.9 for the
> Povidone-iodine gel group and 7244.4 for controls.
> Post-catheterisation values were 44.7 and 658.2,
> respectively.

Types of Infecting Organisms:
Staphylococcus, Streptococcus, Enterococcus,

Time of Urine Sample/UTI (from Catheter insertion):
Bacterial count at 3 minutes post-catheterisation

CAUTI Incidence Rate (as percentage) in:

Intervention Group:

Control Group:

Statistical significance:

> Bacterial count reduction achieved with
> Povidone-iodine lubricating gel was sig-
> nificantly greater than achieved with the
> control lubricating gel.
> Statistical analysis, using the Mann-
> Whitney U-test, giving the value of $p<0.02$

UTI Rate according to Gender: All male subjects

𝔽 **Figure 9.1** Fay's data extraction forms.

Practice session 9.1

Below we have included a number of templates that you might want to use for your
own data extraction (Boxes 9.3 to 9.7).

Box 9.3   Template to use for quantitative generic data extraction

Details of study 1 (bibliographical reference):

Title:

Source:

Purpose of the study:

Reviewer's name: Date:

Study design:

Population:

Sample size:

Criteria of diagnosis:

Any secondary diagnosis:

Exclusion criteria:

Setting:

Intervention:

Comparative intervention:

Outcomes:

Adverse effects:

Box 9.4   Template to use for qualitative generic data extraction

Date of data extraction:

Reviewer:

Bibliographical details of study:

Purpose of study:

Study design:

Setting:

Population:

Sample selection:

Number:

Age:

Education, years:

Ethnicity/race:

Religion:

Relationship of family member:

Primary diagnosis at time of event:

Exposure:

Box 9.5 Outcomes: theme 1				
Population experiences 1				
Page	Col.	Line	Data extracted	Subthemes

Box 9.6 Outcomes: theme 2				
Population experiences 2				
Page	Col.	Line	Data extracted	Subthemes

Box 9.7 Outcomes: theme 3				
Population experiences 3				
Page	Col.	Line	Data extracted	Subthemes

Key points

- Data extraction involves going back to the primary articles and highlighting the relevant information that will answer the research question.
- This involves extracting data related to the population included, the intervention, comparative group and particularly the outcomes (the PICO components).
- To standardize this process and improve the validity of the results, it is crucial to compile a data extraction form.

Summary

This chapter discussed the third stage of the method of review associated with how to extract the appropriate qualitative and quantitative data from your research papers. The importance of using a form or framework to standardize and increase the reliability and validity for all stages of the process was clarified by using relevant examples from nursing practice.

Question and Answer (Q&A)

(Q) Are there any standardized data extraction forms or frameworks available to aid with data extraction for both quantitative and qualitative reviews?

(A) There are several data extraction frameworks available both on the internet as well as in numerous research methods books and systematic review websites. However, as the data extraction form is generally designed to a very specific research or review question it is unlikely that you will find a data extraction form that answers your own specific review question. Having said that, looking at other data extraction forms both in your specific area and in other areas (for example on the internet or in other students' dissertations) may help you with the general design of your own data extraction form. We would also recommend that prior to commencing your own systematic literature review you should also explore what is available in the literature (and elsewhere) and then select the most appropriate ways that these tools could help you complete your own review.

10

Synthesizing, summarizing and presenting your findings

Overview

- Issues to consider when synthesizing and summarizing your results
- Tools to use when synthesizing and summarizing your results
- How and where to get started on presenting your results
- Presenting the results of your search
- Presenting the results of the studies selected based on the title and abstract
- Presenting the results of the studies selected based on reading the full paper
- Presenting a summary of all your included studies
- Presenting a summary of all the critiques of your included papers using the appropriate frameworks
- Presenting a summary of the data extracted (including a synthesis of the overall results)
- Summarizing, synthesizing and presenting your interventions and comparative interventions
- Summarizing, synthesizing and presenting your outcomes
- Summarizing, synthesizing and presenting quantitative outcome measures
- Summarizing, synthesizing and presenting qualitative outcome measures

Issues to consider when synthesizing and summarizing your results

When synthesizing and summarizing your data, there are a number of issues that you need to consider. Popay et al. (2006) state that, 'the synthesis, *at a minimum*, is a summary of the current state of knowledge in relation to a particular review question' (Popay et al. 2006: 6, original emphasis). This is the section where you will attempt to find the answer to your review question. In a quantitative review, if the results are similar enough – for example if the interventions, designs and outcomes are all alike – it may be possible to conduct a statistical procedure, such as a meta-analysis, to combine the results. In a qualitative review the combined results of all the included studies can be synthesized under major themes or subthemes. This is sometimes called a meta-synthesis or meta-ethnography. It involves a similar approach to the methods of qualitative data analysis used in the primary qualitative studies being synthesized (Noyes et al. 2008).The Centre for Reviews and Dissemination (University of York,

2008) suggests that irrespective of what type of data you have extracted, it is important to first undertake a narrative synthesis of the results of your findings to help you
decide what other methods are appropriate.

Practical Tip

In our opinion this is one of the most exciting parts of the review as it is where you
start finding out the answer to your review question.

Popay et al. (2006) state:

> Narrative synthesis is a form of storytelling…bringing together evidence in a way
> that tells a convincing story of why something needs to be done, or needs to be
> stopped, or why we have no idea whether a long established policy or practice
> makes a positive difference is one of the ways in which the gap between research,
> policy and practice can start to be bridged. Telling a trustworthy story is at the
> heart of narrative synthesis.

(Popay et al. 2006: 5)

Popay et al. (2006) have provided some excellent guidance on synthesizing data and
have described some specific tools and techniques that can be used when synthesizing
your results. They suggest that narrative synthesis may be used in a number of different ways.

- Before undertaking a specialist approach, such as statistical meta-analysis or
  meta-ethnography.
- Instead of a specialist synthesis approach, because the studies included are insufficiently similar to allow for this.
- When the review question dictates the inclusion of a wide range of research
  designs including qualitative and quantitative designs (Popay et al. 2006: 7).

Recapping briefly from Chapter 7 once you have selected your papers, appraised the
quality of your papers and extracted the appropriate data, how do you go about synthesizing (or combining) the results obtained from all the primary papers you have
included? Some of the key points associated with data extraction can be summarized
as follows.

- Are the data sufficiently similar?
- Are there caveats (explanations to prevent misinterpretation) that need to be
  acknowledged?
- Are there any particular trends or themes?
- Does the data seem to point in one direction or several?

In many disciplines, however, such as nursing and the social sciences, the quantitative
studies involved are either significantly different or in many cases involve qualitative
studies that require different methods of synthesis. Some reviews may also include

studies of different designs (mixed methods). Irrespective of the type of review, there will still need to be some form of summary or synthesis.

Although the primary aim of a review is to answer a clinical question and alter practice, it is important to write up the systematic literature review and publish it so that other nurses can benefit from the findings. Depending on whether the systematic literature review is being conducted for a dissertation or is being written up for journal publication, different results may be presented depending on the submission requirements. Journal articles and the Cochrane Library usually have their own recommendations or criteria for presenting the results.

Tools to use when synthesizing and summarizing your results

There are numerous tools that you can use to summarize, synthesize and present your data. A few of the most common ones are listed below.

- Textual descriptions, which means written words that everyone is familiar with.
- Grouping of similar data, for example tabulation (presenting the results in tables).
- Transforming data into a common rubric (name of a particular group or section), for example changing actual numbers from different papers into percentages.
- Charts, which can include histograms, pie-charts and others.
- Translating data either by a thematic or content analysis (Popay et al. 2006).

Practical Tip

We recommend that prior to commencing the review you look at the various tools and checklists available to find one that best suits you and your review.

How and where to get started on presenting your results

This section discusses how to go about summarizing, synthesizing and presenting your results. There are a number of different ways you can do this. The methods for summarizing and synthesizing your data discussed within this book are primarily aimed at the novice reviewer. For more experienced reviewers, the PRISMA (Preferred Reporting Items for Systematic Reviews and Meta-Analyses) document outlines how systematic reviews should be reported for academic journals (http://www.prisma-statement.org/) (Moher et al. 2009).

Essentially the results of everything you have done so far need to be presented, including:

1 Presenting the results of your search.
2 Presenting the results of the studies selected based on the title and abstract.
3 Presenting the results of the studies selected based on reading the full paper.
4 Presenting a summary of all your included studies.
5 Presenting a summary of all the critiques of the included papers using the appropriate frameworks.
6 Presenting a summary of the data extracted (including a synthesis of the overall results).

All the above will now be discussed in turn below.

1. Presenting the results of your search

The results of the comprehensive search can be presented either textually or in a table. When writing the search up, it is important to identify all the databases that you have searched and the results you found, so that anyone reading the review can ascertain how comprehensive, transparent and replicable your review is. When presenting the results, it is usual to include the databases searched with the dates included, the date of the search, the number of hits, the number of articles discarded and the number of articles left that need to be reviewed by title and abstract. Results presented in tables also need to be explained fully. Table 10.1 provides an example of how the results of your systematic literature review in nursing could be presented.

Table 10.1 An example of one way of presenting the results of the systematic search

Database with dates	Search date	Number of hits retrieved from the search	Number of articles discarded because of irrelevant titles	Number of articles duplicated from another database	Number of articles to be reviewed by title and abstract
CINAHL (2000–2015)	20/11/15	1569	1456	79	34
MEDLINE (1963–2015)	21/11/15	1847	1346	244	284
EMBASE (1996–2015)	23/11/15	2485	1567	600	318

Practice session 10.1

For your own review question, using the template (Box 10.1), try to fill in the databases you used when searching for your own review question. Write down the dates included, the date of the search, the number of hits, the number of articles discarded and the number of articles remaining that need to be reviewed by title and abstract. As mentioned in Chapter 6 you can now see how important it is to document all your searches. If you don't do this, it will mean that you will need to conduct the search again.

---

2. Presenting the results of the studies selected based on the title and abstract

Once the search of a review is conducted, the second step of the systematic literature review is the selection of the primary research studies that meet your inclusion criteria, based on reading the abstracts and titles. Table 10.2 is an example of one way these results could be presented. The first three columns have been filled in to illustrate this

Box 10.1 Template to use for presenting the results of your systematic search

Database with dates	Search date	Number of hits retrieved from search	Number of articles discarded due to irrelevant titles	Number of articles duplicated from another database	Number of articles to be reviewed by title and abstract
CINAHL					
MEDLINE					
EMBASE					
COCHRANE					
AMED					

point. In column 1 the action is to include the paper as all the criteria have been met. In column 2 the action is to exclude the paper as two of the criteria have not been met. In column 3 the action is to read the full paper before deciding whether to include or exclude the study as it is unclear from reading the abstract whether or not advocacy was included in the primary paper under consideration.

3. Presenting the results of the studies selected based on reading the full paper

The third step involves presenting the results of the studies included based on reading the full paper and can be presented in a similar format. The final action in this stage is now to include or exclude the paper. Presenting a table similar to that in Table 10.2 will enable the reader to know precisely on which selection criteria you based your decision to select your papers. It makes the process of how you conducted your systematic review very clear, transparent and replicable. Remember to include the bibliographic

Table 10.2 An example of one way of presenting the results of the included studies based on reading the title and abstract

Abstract number	1	2	3	4	5
Population					
Women?	√	√	√		
Over 18?					
Intervention					
Advocacy	√	√	?		
Comparative group					
Peer groups or general practice treatment?	√	×	√		
Outcomes					
Women's experiences of interventions?	√	×	√		
Type of study					
Phenomenological	√	√	√		
*Action	Include	Exclude	Read full article		

*Include (read full article); exclude; read full article.

details of the full articles (i.e. the names of the authors, the titles of the articles and the journals they were published in etc.) so the reader can know exactly which papers were included and which were excluded and why.

Practice session 10.2

Now use one of the templates provided to present the inclusion results of the criteria you used for your review. You should already have done this in Chapter 5. Please note that for the first phase of the selection of studies, your actions can be to include, exclude or read the full paper and then make a decision (Box 10.2). For the second phase where you read the full paper, your decision can only be to include or exclude (Box 10.3). Whatever type of review question you have (i.e. either PICO or PEO), the results of the two stages you undertook to select your papers should be presented.

---

4. Presenting a summary of all your included studies

The fourth step is to provide a summary and present a description of all the primary studies you included within your systematic literature review. Ideally, the details of what is presented should be the same for each study. Tables 10.3 and 10.4 show two

Box 10.2   Template for you to use for presenting the results of the included studies based on reading the title and abstract and using the PICO format

Abstract number	1	2	3	4	5
Population					
Intervention					
Comparative group					
Outcomes					
Type of study					
*Action: include or read full article or exclude					

Box 10.3   Template for you to use for presenting the results of the included studies on reading the full paper and using the PEO format

Paper number	1	2	3	4	5
Population					
Exposure					
Outcomes					
Type of study					
*Action: include or exclude					

examples of how information could be presented in tabular format. In Table 10.3 the first row is filled in as an example of the details that could be included for one study using Mary's case study as an example. In Table 10.4 you can see an example of what one of Sue's paper summaries on witnessed resuscitation could look like. In both versions, the information relating to all components of PICO or PEO need to be provided.

There is another way to present the details for all your included studies and that is simply to write a narrative summary with structured headings (similar to an abstract). If you choose to write it out this way, make sure that you include all the details relating to the population, intervention or exposure and outcomes.

M **Table 10.3** An example of how Mary could describe one study that she included in her review based on all components of the PICO structure

Study	Population	Intervention	Comparative intervention	Outcomes
1. Jones, M. and Smith, L. (2006) Effect of advocacy compared to usual care on women's quality of life. *Clinical Nursing* 20 (1): 56–60	Sample selection: Volunteers recruited from advertisements posted in various Community agencies Number: 24 Mean age: 24 years old, range 21–51 years Abusive relationship status: 45% were currently in abusive relationships with no intention of leaving, 35% were trying to leave abusive relationships	60% in individual counselling or a domestic violence support group	40% usual care	Quality of life (QOL) scales Advocacy group pre-intervention QOL values: 30/50 (50 is the average figure for QOL for healthy individuals) Post-intervention QOL values: QOL value 40/50 Usual care group pre-intervention: QOL value 29/50 Post-intervention usual care group: QOL value 30/50 (no difference in QOL post-treatment)

S **Table 10.4** An example of how Sue could describe one of her qualitative studies using the PEO framework

Paper 2 Full bibliographic reference	O'Brien, J. and Fothergill-Bourbonnais, F. (2004) The experience of trauma resuscitation in the Emergency Department: Themes from seven patients. Journal of Emergency Nursing 30 (3): 216–224.
Population	Four men and three women over the age of 18. Four patients were involved in motor vehicle collisions and three suffered falls.
Exposure	The lived experience of patients undergoing resuscitation with and without family presence.
Outcome	Gain an insight of the experiences of patients undergoing resuscitation as shaped by the context of their circumstances.
Results	Four main themes emerged: recollection, confidence in staff, lack of knowledge and experience of being a patient and survival. These main themes consisted of numerous threads: frustration, feeling scared, pain free, kept patients well informed, lack of knowledge and experience of being a patient, tone of voice was calm and soothing, feeling safe, organized and caring, male patients thought family members got in the way, female patients felt that family members' presence was a source of comfort and reassurance, feeling important and comforted, going to get out, appreciation for life, positivity and vulnerability.

Practice session 10.3

Select the appropriate template (Boxes 10.4 and 10.5) for your own review question and try to fill in the details of your own included studies.

Box 10.4   Template to use for describing your included studies (PEO format)

Study	Population	Intervention	Comparative intervention	Outcomes
1				
2				
3				
4				
5				

---

5. Presenting a summary of all the critiques of your included papers using the appropriate frameworks

In the fifth step, the summary of the results of your critiques can be presented in either tabular or narrative format. When presenting the results of your critiques, it is worth critiquing each study individually and then presenting a shortened version of the answers to all the critique questions for all the studies you included in one comprehensive table. This will likely run into a number of pages. Presenting the overall results of all your critiques in this way shows that you have appropriately and methodically critiqued the research papers included within your review. Presenting the results of your critiques in this way is helpful when you come to discuss your review

Box 10.5   Template to use for describing your included studies in another way (PICO format)

Study	Population	Intervention	Comparative intervention	Outcomes
1				
2				
3				
4				
5				

(see Chapter 11). Table 10.5 shows a hypothetical example for answering only the first five questions for a paper using Caldwell's critical appraisal framework (Caldwell et al. 2011). Presenting the results in this way is helpful when discussing your results later in your review.

Although some critical appraisal frameworks, for example the Caldwell and McMaster frameworks, do not yield a numerical value of the quality of the paper, for the purposes of your own systematic review it is still possible to assign values either for the overall paper quality or for each appraisal question based on your subjective appraisal. A Likert scale can be made up representing the values of one through to five, with one representing a paper of very poor overall quality and five representing a paper of very good overall quality. Alternatively, it is possible to assign a numerical value to each question and then to add up all the individual scores.

The Caldwell framework has 18 questions. For each question you could have three possible answers (numbers) with an answer of no = 0, partly = 1 and yes = 2. The maximum value that any study could get using the Caldwell framework is 36. At this stage, if you plan only to include studies of good or very good quality in your review, it is important that you state a cut-off point. For example, you could state that any studies

Table 10.5 An example of how to present the results for the full methodological quality (critical appraisal) of your included studies based on the Caldwell et al. (2011) framework (first five questions only)

Paper	Q1 Does the title reflect the content?	Q2 Are the authors credible?	Q3 Does the abstract summarize the key components?	Q4 Is the rationale for undertaking the research clearly outlined?	Q5 Is the literature review comprehensive and up-to-date?
1	Yes, the title includes the population, intervention, comparative intervention and outcomes and accurately reflected the content.	Yes, the authors appear credible. The first author has a doctorate in nursing, which shows her competence to conduct research. The other two authors are both registered nurses.	Yes, the abstract was very comprehensive and structured appropriately with all sections included.	Yes, the rationale for conducting the study was very clear. The authors critiqued all the available literature in the area and very clearly showed the gap in knowledge, which they then proceeded to address.	Yes, a comprehensive literature was provided. All the papers mentioned were also appropriately critiqued.

achieving fewer than 20 points (out of a total of 36 points) will be excluded from your review. Alternatively you could include all the studies (even the poor ones) and then conduct a separate analysis to assess whether the poor studies significantly affected the overall results of your review.

Practice session 10.4

For your own review use one of the templates (Boxes 10.6 and 10.7) based on the Caldwell et al. (2011) framework to critique your papers. You may have already done this when you critiqued each paper individually, so it should now be a simple matter of cutting and pasting the answers from your individual critique to the template. This will allow you to see the results of all the critiques you undertook in a collated format. If your original individual critiques are too long, you can cut and paste only the most important and relevant information. The two templates are similar. The main difference is that the Box 10.6 template does not include a numerical value for each question, whereas the Box 10.7 template does. If you decide to use Box 10.6, you can still rate your paper from one (very poor) through to five (very good) as discussed above.

---

6. Presenting a summary of the data extracted (including a synthesis of the overall results)

Whatever your review question, in the final step the data you extracted will need to include details related to the population, interventions, comparative interventions (or

Box 10.6   Template to use for presenting your summary of the results of the full methodological quality (critical appraisal) of your included studies based on the Caldwell et al. (2011) framework (first five questions only)

Paper	Q1 Does the title reflect the content?	Q2 Are the authors credible?	Q3 Does the abstract summarize the key components?	Q4 Is the rationale for undertaking the research clearly outlined?	Q5 Is the literature review comprehensive and up-to-date?
1					
2					
3					
4					
5					

exposures) and outcomes of all the primary studies you decided to include within your review. All these will now be discussed in turn.

Extracting data relevant to your population group

The way that data extracted from your studies are synthesized and presented depends on the type of data being handled. If you have quantitative data, the usual method is to present them either in tabular format or as a chart. If you have qualitative data, it is usual to present them in themes and subthemes in a similar way to how the results of a primary qualitative study are presented. With regard to presenting the details related to population groups, ethnicities etc, these data are usually numerical, for example you might say paper 1 had 20 subjects, paper 2 had 40 subjects and so on. If you decide to include the religious affiliation of the populations you are looking at, you may want

Box 10.7   Template to use for presenting your summary of the full methodological quality assessments of your included studies based on the Caldwell et al. (2011) framework, including an overall numerical value

Questions for qualitative studies based on the Caldwell framework		Paper 1	Paper 2	Paper 3
1	Does the title reflect the content?			
2	Are the authors credible?			
	Background and literature review			
3	Does the abstract summarize the key components?			
4	Is the rationale for undertaking the research clearly outlined?			
5	Is the literature review comprehensive and up-to-date?			
6	Is the aim of the research clearly stated?			
7	Are all ethical issues identified and addressed?			
	Methods			
8	Is the methodology identified and justified?			
9	Are the philosophical background and study design identified and the rationale for choice of design evident?			
10	Are the major concepts identified?			
11	Is the context of the study outlined?			
12	Is selection of participants described and the sample method identified?			
13	Is the method of data collection auditable?			
	Data analysis			
14	Is the method of data analysis credible and confirmable?			
	Results			
15	Are the results presented in a way that is appropriate and clear?			
16	Are the results transferable?			
	Discussion			
17	Is the discussion comprehensive?			
	Conclusions and implications			
18	Is the conclusion comprehensive?			
	Numerical assessment awarded by author (maximum score is 36 points)	__/36		

to consider using something like a pie chart or histogram. Table 10.6, Figure 10.1 and Figure 10.2 are examples of how you could present the number of subjects in each study. Charts and tables can be used to synthesize and present the population numbers in both qualitative and quantitative reviews.

Table 10.6 Number of participants in all the primary studies included in your review

Article	Number of subjects
Jones (1988)	40
Davies (1992)	60
Smith (2005)	70
Bettany (2008)	80

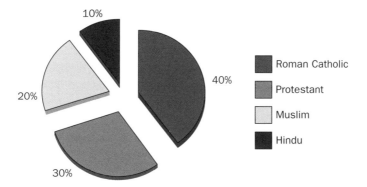

Figure 10.1 Religious affiliation for all subjects in all included studies.

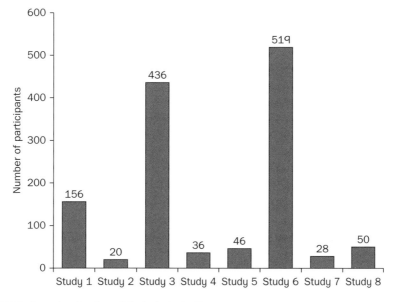

Figure 10.2 Sample size for all included studies.

Summarizing, synthesizing and presenting your interventions and comparative interventions

The types of interventions and comparative interventions used in all your included studies could be combined to produce a pie chart or they could be presented in a table. Table 10.7 illustrates how the percentages of participants in the intervention and control interventions could be presented. The pie chart (Figure 10.3) shows an alternative method that could be used.

Table 10.7 Types of interventions

Type of intervention	Number of subjects
Group advocacy	30%
Individual sessions	10%
Both	10%
Usual care	50%

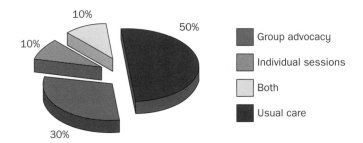

Figure 10.3 Number of subjects in each type of intervention from all included studies.

Summarizing, synthesizing and presenting your outcomes

The summary of the outcomes data extracted depends on the type of data you are handling. If you are synthesizing quantitative data, the usual method is to present the data either in tabular format or as a chart or other alternative graphical format. If they are qualitative data, it is usually easier to present the data through themes and subthemes. It is important when quoting anything to write down exactly where in the primary paper you got this information from (i.e. state the page, column and line numbers) as you will be referring to this later when you discuss them within the discussion section of your review.

Summarizing, synthesizing and presenting quantitative outcome measures

Outcome measures provide the answer to the research question. As with the population and intervention, quality of life scores in Mary's case example could be presented in a table or a graph. Table 10.8 and Figure 10.4 show examples of how Mary could

Ⓜ **Table 10.8** Mean quality of life scores before and after advocacy intervention and usual care for all included studies

Mean quality of life scores for each article as measured by the SF-36 scale

	Advocacy group		Usual care group	
	Before	After	Before	After
Jones (2003)	30/50	40/50	29/50	30/50
Davies (2007)	25/50	38/50	24/50	26/50
Smith (1994)	23/50	41/50	23/50	24/50
Bettany (2008)	21/50	44/50	18/50	17/50

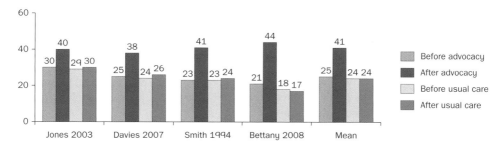

Ⓜ **Figure 10.4** Mean quality of life scores before and after advocacy intervention and usual care for all included studies.

present the combined quality of life scores from all her primary studies, both before and after the interventions.

Summarizing, synthesizing and presenting qualitative outcome measures

Qualitative outcome measures are generally synthesized and presented under themes and subthemes in qualitative primary studies. Presenting qualitative outcomes in systematic literature reviews is no different. Sue could present the outcomes from her qualitative systematic review on witnessed resuscitation in various ways. Sue had three population groups: the patients, the families of the patient and the healthcare professionals. Sue's aim was to appraise their views and perspectives and evaluate any similarities and differences between them that would impact on or change nursing practice. Below are examples of how Sue could synthesize the outcomes from two of her population groups (the patients and the healthcare professionals) under themes and present them in a clear format.

§ Sue found that three main themes emerged from the patients' experiences of resuscitation and invasive procedures, as follows.

- Theme 1: recollection of the resuscitation and survival instinct.
- Theme 2: family presence.
- Theme 3: confidence in staff.

One way Sue could present the qualitative outcomes is presented below.

Theme 1: recollection of the resuscitation and survival instinct. Seven out of ten studies included in this systematic review identified recollections of fear and frustration by the patient during the resuscitation event, which changed when they saw or heard the voice of a family member. During their family members' presence, the patients felt less alone, and more loved and supported. The extracts below illustrate this:

> I was very scared. I thought I would never have a leg again. I thought I might die. I remember waking up and seeing all those doctors. I was like, Where am I? Something is wrong! I looked over and saw my dad and my mother. They were there to help me, to hold my hand, to give me a hug.
>
> (Eichhorn et al. (2001) page 51, col. 1, lines 22–28)

> It would have been awful to be there alone and have no family there by your side. I was scared that the lumbar puncture was going to hurt. I was afraid. Having him [my dad] there was so comforting.
>
> (Eichhorn et al. (2001) page 52, col. 1, lines 1–10)

Theme 2: family presence. Five out of ten studies also highlighted the importance of family presence, which was a key motivational factor in the patients' belief that they would get out of the A&E department and return to pre-injury life.

> When I knew I was OK – and it's hard to tell why I knew it, but I knew the moment that they started coming around and checking me, I knew that I was going to be okay. I knew it with a surety, especially when I saw my mum and dad were beside me and would be there to help me recover.
>
> (O'Brien and Fothergill-Bourbonnais (2004) page 221, col. 2, lines 17–32)

Theme 3: confidence in staff. Six out of ten papers showed that patients had great confidence (trust and faith) in the medical professionals. The extracts below highlight very clearly the strong support and admiration for the healthcare team when the patients sensed and received comfort from the staff and were kept well informed of the procedures that they (patients) were undergoing.

> They warned me there was going to be lots of staff and not to be concerned . . . I felt they were treating me as if I were important.
>
> (O'Brien and Fothergill-Bourbonnais (2004) page 221, col. 1, lines 19–24)

They always kept me informed . . . that's a very positive reassurance for me that I was part of the team getting me better.

(O'Brien and Fothergill-Bourbonnais (2004) page 220, col. 2, lines 5–11)

For healthcare professionals' experiences of resuscitation and/or invasive procedures, Sue could report the themes and extracts from her data extraction and synthesis of the professionals' perceptions as follows. Sue found that two main themes emerged from healthcare professionals' experiences of resuscitation and invasive procedures.

- Theme 1: judgement call.
- Theme 2: threat to comfort zone of healthcare professionals.

Sue could illustrate these two themes in the following way.

Theme 1: judgement call. All the primary qualitative papers identified issues relating to staff having to decide whether the situation was viable for family member presence.

And what is more important, giving the person the right drug or trying to walk around family? I think space is the issue here.

(Timmermans (1997) page 158, col. 1, lines 4–5)

The perceived lack of medical knowledge of the patient's family by the medical staff also contributed to healthcare professionals' decisions as to whether to include or exclude the relatives, as can be seen from the following extract.

As a layperson, I think it adds insult to injury because there are so many traumatic things that happen therapeutically from a medical perspective but could be perceived as additional trauma.

(Knott and Kee (2005) page 195, col. 1, lines 30–45)

Theme 2: threat to comfort zone of healthcare professionals. Another theme which surfaced within all the papers was the challenge that family presence presented to healthcare professionals during the resuscitation or invasive procedure. Family members being present within the resuscitation room made staff question their confidence in their own skills, thus contributing to stressful outcomes for staff as they attempted to do their job. This is clearly seen from the following two extracts.

OK, let's face it, this is why it makes us uncomfortable. When we are doing resuscitations, we are off… it is a mechanical thing. We don't want it to be just a mechanical thing, we want it to be a caring thing and yet we want to remain emotionally aloof so that we can feel that we can function better. We certainly don't want to ever make mistakes in front of a family member. You mix up the drug boxes sometimes. Sometimes you forget to take off a tourniquet…Sometimes these things happen. You don't want to ever have a family see you make a mistake in resuscitation. For the family member that is just terrible. You don't want to have something go wrong – an IV gets pulled out accidentally.

(Timmermans (1997) page 158, col. 1, lines 29–40)

But you do feel like you're on stage, like somebody's watching your performance. But I'm pretty comfortable with my knowledge and skills, so it doesn't really bother me to have somebody there, I just have a heightened awareness…You know, we have to show the family that we're doing absolutely everything that we can do, and you start to feel like you're not benefitting the patient, you're actually increasing their suffering.

(Knott and Kee (2005) page 196, col. 2, lines 24–39)

Accompanying these thoughts, another excerpt highlighted concerns that as the healthcare professionals were conducting their job in an effort to sustain life, they may have appeared insensitive in their manner while conducting the resuscitation and this is viewed as being cautious and reflecting on their practice in a judgemental manner, a manner that the relatives may see as not treating their loved one in a caring manner but treating them as if they were 'a person with a condition'.

'With every patient you just log on, do your work and that's it. It's not Mr So-and-so. It is a patient, a person with an aortic aneurysm, it's a person with bilateral femoral fractures, it is not a patient with a name and that'. When discussing being present during the resuscitation of their family member, the HCP [healthcare professional] answered negatively, ' . . . . you are going to be in the way because you are emotionally involved'.

(Goodenough and Brysiewicz (2003) pages 60–61, cols 2, 1, lines 24–39 and 1–5)

The extracts from both the patients' perspectives and the healthcare professionals' perspectives illustrate that some of their views are similar: both parties are aware of the patients' needs but a number of their perspectives differ significantly. Although the patients feel comforted by the presence of their family members, healthcare professionals are not always comfortable with this and sometimes feel that the relatives get in the way. These similarities and contrasting views will provide very good material for Sue to consider in her discussion section.

Practice session 10.5

If your own review question is qualitative, try writing out the main themes and selecting the most appropriate extracts from the data you extracted in Chapter 9.

🔑 Key points

- The synthesis is a summary of the current state of knowledge in relation to a particular review question.
- In a quantitative review, if the results are similar enough, it may be possible to conduct a statistical procedure, such as a meta-analysis, to combine the results.

- In a qualitative review, the combined results of all the included studies can be synthesized under major themes or subthemes. This is sometimes called a meta-synthesis or meta-ethnography.

- Irrespective of what type of data you have extracted, it is important to always undertake a narrative synthesis of the results of your findings to help you decide what other methods are appropriate.

- Narrative synthesis is a form of storytelling.

- Narrative synthesis may be used in a number of different ways, including the following:

  - before undertaking a specialist approach such as a statistical meta-analysis or meta-ethnography

  - instead of a specialist synthesis approach because the studies included are insufficiently similar

  - when the review question includes a wide range of different research designs including qualitative and quantitative designs.

- The key points associated with the data extracted to some review questions can be summarized as follows.

  - Are the data sufficiently similar?

  - Are there caveats (explanations to prevent misinterpretation) that need to be acknowledged?

  - Are there any particular trends or themes?

  - Do the data seem to point in one direction or several?

- There are numerous tools that you can use to summarize, synthesize and present your data; some of the more common ones include:

  - textual descriptions

  - grouping of similar data

  - transforming data into a common rubric

  - charts

  - translating data either by a thematic or content analysis.

- The results of everything you did in your review needs to be presented:

  - the results of your search

  - the results of the studies you selected based on the title and abstract

  - the results of your included studies based on reading the full paper

  - a summary of all your included studies

  - a summary of all the papers you critiqued

  - a summary of the data extracted (including a synthesis of the overall results).

Summary

This chapter discussed the issues that you need to consider when summarizing, synthesizing and presenting the results of your quantitative or qualitative systematic literature review in nursing practice. A narrative synthesis needs to be included for whatever type of data you have extracted. This can be done by using a number of different tools to summarize, organize and condense your data. The results of all the methods you have undertaken within your review need to be presented. A key point when summarizing, synthesizing and presenting your results is to make sure that you present everything in a clear, transparent and easy to understand format.

Question and Answer (Q&A)

(Q) Does it matter how you present your results?

(A) It is important to present your findings in ways that best represent the type of review you have undertaken. For example, figures, tables, charts for quantitative and narrative or extracts for a qualitative review.

11

Writing up your discussion and completing your review

Overview

- Structuring the discussion of your systematic literature review
- Summarizing your findings in words
- Discussing all the results you presented in the previous section
  - Discussing the search results
  - Discussing the results of the studies selected based on the title and abstract and the results of the included studies based on reading the full paper
  - Discussing the studies included in your review
  - Discussing the quality of your included studies in a synthesized format
  - Discussing the data extracted (including a synthesis of the overall results)
- Developing and/or discussing the theory on how the intervention or exposure works
- Comparing and contrasting the findings of your study
- Relating the findings back to the objectives set out and the initial area of interest
- Pointing to any methodological shortcomings
- Discussing the ethical aspects of the included studies
- Discussing the findings with respect to practice
- Revealing questions for future research on this topic
- Stating some overall conclusions about the study
- Writing up your systematic literature review
- Academic writing skills: tips on style, grammar and syntax

Structuring the discussion of your systematic literature review

Docherty and Smith (1999) state:

> Structure is the most difficult part of writing, no matter whether you are writing a novel, a play, a poem, a government report, or a scientific paper. If the structure is right then the rest can follow fairly easily, but no amount of clever language can compensate for a weak structure. Structure is important so that readers don't become lost. They should know where they've come from, where they are, and

where they are headed. A strong structure also allows readers to know where to look for particular information and makes it more likely that all important information will be included.

(Docherty and Smith 1999: 1224)

Docherty and Smith (1999) suggest that the structure for scientific papers should include a statement of the principal findings, a discussion of the strengths and weaknesses of the study and its strengths and weaknesses in relation to other studies. The meaning of the study findings, as well as implications for practice for clinicians and policy-makers, need to be discussed. Finally, the discussion section should conclude by highlighting the importance of addressing unanswered questions and putting forward suggestions for future research. How can you apply these suggestions to writing up the discussion section of your own systematic literature review?

To recap, by now you should have reported the findings from your studies clearly and concisely in the results section. The next step is to discuss your findings fully (as described above). As suggested by Docherty and Smith (1999) and by the Centre for Reviews and Dissemination (2008), start your discussion section with a summary of your major findings (in words, not repeating the figures from the previous section). Discuss your findings through comparing and contrasting your results, and then relate your discussion to the background literature. Ensure that you don't just repeat the results section. The easiest way to do this is to discuss each section in the order that you presented them in the results section. Depending on the type of review (qualitative or quantitative) the theoretical frameworks are usually discussed within the discussion section (mainly for quantitative reviews) whereas some authors choose to combine the two (i.e. writing up the results and discussion together in the same section; this is conducted more frequently for qualitative reviews). A summary of the key issues that could be included in the discussion section are listed below and then described in detail.

- Summarizing your findings in words.
- Discussing all the results you presented in the previous section, in the same order that they were presented, including the following:
  - search results
  - results of the studies selected based on the title and abstract and the results of the included studies based on reading the full paper
  - studies included in your review
  - quality of your included studies in a synthesized format
  - data extracted (including a synthesis of the overall results).
- Developing and/or discussing the theory or theories on how the intervention or exposure works.
- Comparing and contrasting the findings of your study.
- Relating the findings back to the objectives set out and the initial area of interest.
- Pointing to any methodological shortcomings.
- Discussing the ethical aspects of the included studies.
- Discussing the findings with respect to practice.
- Revealing questions for future research on this topic.
- Stating some overall conclusions about the study.

Each of the points above will now be discussed using fictitious examples and extracts from the four case studies. A few extracts from the Cochrane Review I participated in are also included (Negrini et al. 2010). Please remember there are a number of ways to do this, each of which will include some or most of the points below. Your discussion needs to be clear, comprehensive and easy for the reader to follow.

Summarizing your findings in words

It is a good idea to start writing your discussion section with a brief summary of the review findings. You could start by discussing the types of research designs that were included.

ℂ For example, Cheryl in her scoliosis study could say something like the following.

> In answer to the review question on the effectiveness of braces for adolescents with idiopathic scoliosis, this review found only six studies that met the strict inclusion criteria. Three of these were randomized controlled studies and three were cohort studies.

Next Cheryl could describe the three RCTs in more detail and briefly remind the reader about the results of these studies.

> One randomized controlled trial (Beaver et al. 2009) compared rigid braces to elastic braces and found low quality evidence in favour of rigid braces. The two randomized controlled trials by Smith et al. (2004) and Thompson et al. (2006) found low quality evidence for the effectiveness of the hard brace versus observation alone. Unfortunately these trials looked at different outcomes and could not, therefore, be combined statistically using a meta-analysis, so the results were synthesized narratively.

Cheryl could also discuss any issues that would allow readers to decide if the results were both applicable and relevant to their own practice:

> The studies included only girls, were all written in English and included only the angle of curvature as an outcome. None of the studies looked at outcomes that were important to the patient such as disability, back pain, quality of life and psychological factors.

In other words if the readers of Cheryl's review were nurse practitioners living in Russia where they had mainly male patients and whose main problems were increased pain and a poor quality of life, they would realize that these results would not be applicable to their practice. Cheryl could also qualify her findings by stating that as there were only a small number of studies, the results 'need to be interpreted with caution'.

Discussing all the results you presented in the previous section

All the results presented in the previous section should be discussed in the same order they were presented there.

Discussing the search results

The search results are usually discussed only briefly. You will already have presented details of your comprehensive search in the results section so there is no need to repeat that.

Practical Tip

What is most important when discussing this section is to highlight any issues of the search process that may have adversely affected your search results and produced biased results.

For example, did you search only English-language journals? Was your search truly comprehensive? For example, did you include hand searching of all relevant literature as well as a thorough search for all the grey literature (PhD theses, conference proceedings) relevant to the review question? Did you actually contact any key people in the field to find out whether or not they had further publications in the field? In summary, this is where you highlight what you have or have not done and how this may have introduced any bias in the results of your search. For example, Cheryl could say something like the following:

> A comprehensive search was conducted to retrieve papers that would answer the review question and as a result of reading 90 papers' titles and abstracts, only 20 papers that met the strict inclusion criteria were found. Five papers were then excluded as a result of having read the full papers for the following reasons...
> [here Cheryl would state what the reasons were]
> and searching papers that were not available electronically was undertaken as well as searching for conference abstracts and PhD dissertations that were available in electronic format. Key people in the field of scoliosis were emailed to ask if they had any unpublished literature that could be included within the review. No documents were obtained. A factor that could have caused bias in paper selection was that the search was restricted only to English-language papers and so will have excluded any primary papers in other languages.

Discussing the results of the studies selected based on the title and abstract and the results of the included studies based on reading the full paper

The subject of this section should only be briefly discussed. Again, any key issues should be highlighted. If you only selected 3 or 4 papers out of a total of 50 or more original papers, it is necessary to provide a rationale for this. Maybe your inclusion criteria were too rigid, or perhaps you decided to select a group of participants on which not much had been published. It is important to discuss the papers that were excluded and the reasons for this in more detail so that the reader can understand why you excluded any potentially relevant papers.

Discussing the studies included in your review

In this section you need to provide a discussion of the common (or uncommon) features of all the studies that you included. The easiest way to do this is to go through the summary or description tables of your included studies and then proceed to discuss each part of the PICO or PEO components individually. For example, if you considered the population group of all your included studies, you could discuss how many patients in all were included within the review; were they small or large samples? If the total populations of all your included studies amounted to a very small number, can you really generalize your results? How old were the participants? Did some studies have much older patients whereas some of them included only very young ones? Could these have had an adverse impact on the outcomes of your results? Were all the studies included conducted within the same type of healthcare setting? If some studies were conducted in a tertiary care setting and others were conducted in care homes, this would let the reader know that the settings were quite diverse. Were all the interventions and comparative interventions exactly the same? If not, how did they differ? Were the outcomes evaluated in all your included studies the same and if not how did this impact on your ability to synthesize the results? All the above are examples of questions that could be discussed depending on your specific review question. Here is an extract from Sue's case study on witnessed resuscitation:

§ The seven qualitative studies included within this systematic literature review utilized either grounded theory or descriptive phenomenology. These were chosen for this review as they focused on the lived experience of individuals, aiming to gain an in-depth picture of the populations' feelings and perceptions of the phenomena (Holloway and Wheeler 1996: 15). Qualitative research is beneficial to this review and healthcare research because it adopts a holistic (person-centred) approach. A person-centred approach is associated with gaining the overall picture of life context, beliefs and values in the human environment. It is this aspect of the research that becomes a strength of qualitative studies, whereby quantitative methods would be inappropriate as they do not study subjective, humanistic lifestyles (Leininger 1985: 23). As identified by Holloway and Wheeler (2002: 6), quantitative research is useful, although it neglects participants' perspectives within the context of their environment. All the included studies were conducted in a similar setting although the hospitals varied in whether or not they used protocols for witnessed resuscitation. Four out of seven of the studies included the perspectives of the patients and six out of seven the perspectives of the patient, the family and the healthcare professionals.

In Sue's extract, she first provides a rationale for using qualitative research and why this specific methodology is the most appropriate for her review question. Sue clarifies the strengths of qualitative research for evaluating witnessed resuscitation and also explains why quantitative research would not be a suitable methodology. She then goes on to discuss her included papers in more detail.

Discussing the quality of your included studies in a synthesized format

Discussing the quality of your studies is one of the most important aspects of the discussion section and, depending on whether you are planning to write up your results as a report, dissertation or paper, can run into many pages. In Sue's case study, this section will be based on the individual quality appraisals that Sue conducted on each of her studies and which she evaluated earlier on, while conducting her systematic literature review. The key point that Sue needs to remember when writing this section is that the results of all the appraisals of the studies need to be synthesized or combined together to give the reader an *overall summary* of the quality of the papers that were included in the review. This part of the discussion will most likely be one of the longest subsections in the discussion. You will also need to consider whether or not the quality of the included studies affects the outcome of your results. If the methods of a particular study or the study were classed as 'very poor', can you still believe the results and apply them to practice? Obviously you cannot. Here is an extract from Sue's systematic literature review on witnessed resuscitation:

> All papers addressed how the studies ensured trustworthiness. Credibility was heightened in papers by Warren et al. (2006) and Crosby (2009) by utilizing member checking, which is considered the most important technique for establishing credibility according to Lincoln and Guba (1985), whereby the researcher returned to the participants to achieve feedback on interpretation (Polit and Beck 2004: 432). Peer debriefing was also carried out in the papers by Andrews et al. (2005), Willowby et al. (2004) and Bell et al. (2010) as the researchers involved peers in reviewing different aspects of the inquiry. Data, investigator, theoretical and methodological triangulation was evident in some of the studies, which strengthens credibility.

Discussing the data extracted (including a synthesis of the overall results)

The data extracted included aspects relating to the PICO elements for quantitative studies and the PEO elements for qualitative studies. Once you have synthesized the extracted data, it is important to discuss these data within the discussion section. Below is an extract from the discussion section from one qualitative outcome from Sue's review, which she discusses under a specific theme.

Theme 1: threat to comfort zone and judgement call

Within this theme, several threads emerged relating to feelings from healthcare professionals that family presence put additional strain on the team conducting the resuscitation process and outlines some choices they had to make when deciding whether the family members should be present, depending on the individuals coping ability. This view was supported by a patient in the study conducted by Eichhorn et al. (2001: 53) who was asked his opinion on how family presence could affect the healthcare environment. He disclosed that it was important that family members understand that they should conduct themselves in an appropriate manner but '*It should be decided on a case-by-case basis – who can handle it and who cannot!*' Knott and Kee (2005: 198) concede that they do not facilitate family presence for several reasons (a) lack of space, (b) insufficient staff, and (c) the potential that the above may have on creating psychological problems for the family member.

Here is an extract concerning the quality of life outcome from a Cochrane review on braces (Negrini et al. 2010):

Quality of life
Both rigid and elastic braces caused problems, though different kinds of problems. While the rigid brace caused significantly more problems with heat (85% versus 27%), as well as difficulties with donning and doffing, the patients using the elastic braces had difficulties with toileting (Wong 2008). There is low quality evidence from one RCT (N = 43) that a rigid brace is hotter and more difficult to put on and take off than an elastic one, but an elastic one is difficult to manoeuvre during toileting.

(Negrini et al. 2010: 7)

In both the witnessed resuscitation extract and the brace extract, the key issue to be discussed is stated in the first sentence of the paragraph and then the rest of the paragraph goes on to explain what was stated in the first sentence, thus the first sentence is setting the scene for the rest of the paragraph.

Developing and/or discussing the theory on how the intervention or exposure works

In this section it would be helpful, especially if the results of your review are positive or really important (such as witnessed resuscitation), to discuss the theories on how this intervention may work or how policies governing the witnessed resuscitation protocols could be improved or standardized. In Cheryl's review, she could discuss different people's theories as to how hard braces and soft braces work, and what factors may influence whether they work or not, for example compliance (whether or not the patient wears the brace or not). Sue's review on witnessed resuscitation could discuss the importance of witnessed resuscitation to the patients themselves as well as the family, even though the healthcare staff may find it hinders them to have the family around.

Comparing and contrasting the findings of your study

Comparing your findings with the findings of other reviewers is very important. This places the results of your own review within the context of other research and reviews that have already been carried out. Do your review results support the work of others? Do they contradict them? And, if so, why do you believe this is?

Ⓒ In the case of the scoliosis brace review, Cheryl could compare her results with other narrative and systematic reviews and discuss the similarities and differences in the population groups, interventions and outcomes, as well as any methodological problems of the included studies and suggest explanations for possible similarities as well as differences. Below is an extract from the Cochrane brace review I participated in (and on which Cheryl's example is based) and this compares how our review was similar to and/or different from other reviews. Suggestions and explanations for these were discussed as seen below:

> An 'evidence-based review' (Dolan 2007) looked at totally different outcomes from those considered here: the 'rate of surgery' (failure of treatment) in braced groups ranged between 1.4% and 41%. This paper was based on retrospective comparative studies, and on retrospective and prospective case series results, all of which were excluded from the current review. Furthermore, only papers in English were considered, while those adding exercises to bracing were excluded. It was not possible to obtain a good uniformity of methods and outcomes among the papers...These problems could be overcome following the SRS criteria for bracing studies (Richards 2005). Moreover, excluding papers that add exercises to bracing should not be done in the future, because according to SOSORT [*Society on Scoliosis Orthopaedic and Rehabilitation Treatment*] criteria (Negrini 2009), this is a management criterion to increase compliance. In fact, papers including exercises...report very low surgery rates,...comparable to the best results in the bracing papers reported above.
>
> (Negrini et al. 2010: 9)

Relating the findings back to the objectives set out and the initial area of interest

Relating the findings back to the objectives is an important aspect of the discussion section as the discussion is not a standalone part of the review. Here you need to relate what you found in your results back to your objectives and background section. For example, Cheryl could relate her findings back to her objectives:

> The objective of this study was to evaluate the effectiveness of braces for adolescents with idiopathic scoliosis. The results of this review suggest that there is low evidence for their effectiveness.

Pointing to any methodological shortcomings

Pointing to any methodological shortcomings or flaws in your systematic literature review, and how these may affect the interpretation of the results you have found, is one of the key aspects to include within your discussion. Recommendations on how these shortcomings may be rectified in future studies would also be beneficial. Addressing the limitations of the review enables your readers to judge what parts of the review you could have improved on. Knowing the limitations also allows readers to judge the validity of the results for themselves and how applicable the results may be to their own practice. Here is an example of what Sue could have written for her review on this subject.

§ **Limitations of the systematic review**

Due to the primary papers included within this review having numerous methodological shortcomings, the overall outcomes were compromised. The process of reading the full text papers to assess the methodological quality and the data extraction procedure was conducted alone, which could have given rise to bias.

Discussing the ethical aspects of the included studies

The discussion of the ethical issues within the primary papers that you included within your review is important. If you have evaluated papers that made no mention of any ethical approvals or informed consent of their patients, there is the possibility that the authors conducting the studies might not have considered the issues of informed consent, right to withdrawal etc. As Sue highlights in her systematic literature review, ethical approval by local ethical committees is considered as an indicator of reliability and validity since it ensures that the study complies with professional, ethical and scientific standards (Tingle and Cribb 2002: 278–285). Here is an excellent discussion on the ethical issues within Sue's systematic literature review:

> § As noted by Parahoo (2006: 112), all research studies have individual ethical implications and are sometimes more prominent in one design than another. Importantly, the process of interviewing vulnerable participants – such as those identified within this review – warrants serious ethical consideration. Papers 1, 4 and 5 clearly identify that either verbal or written consent was achieved from the participants and ethical approval obtained from either the Board of Managers within the included hospitals or sponsoring University Review Board. Commendably, paper 4 identified 'beneficence' in providing a 'duty of care' as recommended by the Nursing and Midwifery Council (NMC 2004: 4). The studies all asserted autonomy and confidentiality by issuing a pseudonym to participants and identifying the risks against benefit of exposure prior to the study; they also gave participants the choice to withdraw from the study and access to transcripts. The latter is important in qualitative studies to validate interpretations (Van der Woning 1999: 188).

Discussing the findings with respect to practice

An 'implication for practice' subsection should be included within the discussion section. Improving and enhancing practice is one of the most important reasons for conducting your systematic review. Here is an extract from Sue's review:

> § Due to the nature of this 'subjective phenomenon', unless having been involved in witnessed resuscitation, it is difficult to understand personal choice. Although the studies delivered strong support for witnessed resuscitation, there were also concerns about negative issues. As recognized in the background literature and throughout this research, cultural diversity affects values, beliefs and behaviours relating to health and illness therefore responses will be subjective (Eichhorn et al. 2001: 54). Through awareness of our own capabilities, we as professional individuals can recognize personal perceptions and biases to accept family choice

with respectful autonomy and provide a duty of care (NMC 2004: 4). Through conducting this systematic review it has been identified that further studies should be undertaken to gain knowledge from the patient perspective. One commonality within all the studies except Paper 2 was the recommendation for a protocol especially to deal with the psychosocial requirements of relatives as within Paper 7 attitudes towards family presence changed from negative to positive and further advocates initiating a 'pilot' site so as to provide necessary data to implement change by introducing protocols and education to HCPs and laypersons connected to family presence on a national level in the UK (Hulme 2009).

Revealing questions for future research on this topic

Suggesting areas for future research is a key aspect of any discussion. Include the main points investigated within your review that you would like the reader to remember, highlight what is still not known and include suggestions of the most relevant research that you think should be done to further improve practice in this area.

Stating some overall conclusions about the study

The conclusions of your review should provide a summary of the whole review and re-state the key findings. Extracts from Cheryl's brace review are presented first. Her findings were very similar to those provided by Negrini et al.'s (2010: 9) Cochrane review on braces. An extract from Sue's witnessed resuscitation review conclusion is also provided below.

ℂ Conclusion

Today the only alternative to bracing is the so-called 'wait and see' strategy (i.e. observation and eventual surgery). The scientific evidence is in favour of bracing, but quality is very low . . . any future study should look at patient outcomes (not just radiographic outcomes of scoliosis progression) as well as adverse effects, so that balanced conclusions may be generated.

(Negrini et al. 2010: 9)

𝕊 Conclusion

This systematic review has identified a plethora of views from patients, family members and healthcare practitioners surrounding their individual experiences of family presence during resuscitation and/or invasive procedures. Each group identified their preferences within themes that were explored through rich narration, thus giving an overall impression of trustworthiness, which will contribute to informing practice when utilized with expert clinical judgement. Derogatory attitudes from fellow family and peers when identifying the research aims and objectives around the phenomenon of 'witnessed resuscitation' are recalled by the author. This may be through a lack of knowledge and understanding of the topic area and the complexities involved. On reflection, it would be interesting to find out their opinions of the topic after reading this review, for it is important that all individuals are given the choice to be present or not, as in reminiscence, we are all invited to be present at the birth of our loved ones; therefore should we not be included in their departure from life? The ability to understand this particular phenomenon can lead to nursing care that is responsive to the complex experiences of the life world within the resuscitation room. Supported by protocols such as those developed by the Emergency Nurses Associations (ENA 2001: Appendix 4), practitioners can deliver truly holistic care. Until such time, family presence will continue to be highly debated until protocols are institutionalized to aid the decision-making process through relevant evidence-based care (Hulme 2009).

Writing up your systematic literature review

The final step in conducting your systematic literature review is writing it up to a high standard. Depending on why you are conducting your systematic literature review, you may need to write up a dissertation, a journal article, a hospital report or a paper for a commissioning body. Irrespective of where you are planning to write up your review, it is important to take as much care in writing it up as in conducting the review. The report should include all aspects of the systematic review process including the background, objectives, inclusion and exclusion criteria, methods of selecting and appraising your papers, extracting relevant data, the results section, the discussion and conclusions.

As discussed earlier, by the time you have written up the plan or protocol of your review, you should already have the first five major sections written up, albeit in the future tense.

Practical Tip

Once you have completed your review, having the protocol or plan written up makes completing the review much easier as you will not be starting from scratch. In fact the first five sections or chapters of your systematic review should be mostly written up within the protocol (1. Background, 2. Selection criteria, 3. Objectives, 4. Search strategy and 5. Methods). Once you have actually finished your review the aspects of the review that you will need to concentrate on, at this point, are the background section or chapter and making sure it is sufficiently in-depth. You will of course also need to write up and present all your results and discussion sections. Obviously you will also need to go back through your whole systematic review paper or thesis to make sure that you have appropriately and fully written up all the sections of your literature review. In the last chapter (Chapter 12) we have included a checklist in order for you to do so.

Practical Tip

Another important point to consider are the tenses to use when you are writing both the protocol and the full literature review. When writing your protocol or plan you will need to use the future tense as this is something you plan on doing in the very near future. However, when you complete you review it is crucial that you now change all the tenses to the past tense as the review is now completed.

You will need to go back to your plan and update the background section (there may have been more papers or relevant reviews published by this time). You should already have your objectives, inclusion and exclusion criteria, methods for selecting and appraising your papers and data extracting written up, although it will be worth checking them over to ensure you did what you said you would do in your original plan. You should now have only two major sections to write up – the results and the discussion sections, including the conclusion.

It is important to ensure that your report is written up clearly and with great attention to detail, similar to the writing up of a scientific paper. It needs to contain enough detail so other nurses or researchers can replicate your review just by reading through it. The literature suggests that poor quality reporting of primary papers affects readers' ability to interpret the results. Many reports suggest that reviews (as well as intervention papers) often omit crucial details about the interventions or methods of the review, thereby limiting the ability of clinicians and readers of the systematic literature review to evaluate the findings and limiting clinicians' ability to implement the findings in practice (Cochrane Effective Practice and Organisation of Care 2011). Ideally, similar to the writing up of your discussion section, it is best to structure the presentation of your review. Box 11.1 suggests how to present all the sections in the write up of your report.

Academic writing skills: tips on style, grammar and syntax

Many people assume that any literate person can write a research proposal and or systematic review. This is not quite accurate. It is one thing to write a letter or an email to a friend when you go on holiday but quite another matter when it comes to writing in an academic style.

> ### Practical Tip
>
> Writing is a complex skill to master and the only way that most people improve their writing skills is through practice, perseverance and dedication. Most students that I have supervised need to rewrite their paper or dissertation a number of times before it is of an acceptable quality for publication.

When writing up your report it is important to make sure your writing style is in the correct tense. Before completing your report, try to check the spelling, grammar and syntax. Reading a systematic literature review that is full of spelling errors is off-putting and gives the impression that the review was done carelessly and without attention to detail. The following are some tips to help you write up your review and help with your academic writing:

Tips for writing up

- If you are stuck and have writer's block, try using mind mapping exercises or brainstorming with colleagues.
- If possible, try to structure your work in advance.

Box 11.1   Suggested structure of a systematic literature review

Title

Acknowledgements

Abstract

Contents page

Abbreviations or glossary (if relevant)

Structured abstract

- Background

- Objectives

- Search strategy

- Study selection

- Study appraisal

- Data extraction and synthesis

- Results

- Discussion

- Conclusions

Main text

1 Background

2 Review question(s)

3 Objectives

4 Search strategy

5 Study selection

6 Study appraisal

7 Data extraction and synthesis

8 Results

9 Discussion

10 References

11 Conclusions

12 Appendices

- Know what you want to convey before trying to write it.
- Every sentence should contain one idea only.
- Each sentence should follow logically from the one before. A well-written text is a chain of ideas.
- When you write a new paragraph, introduce the main idea of the paragraph in the first line of the paragraph and then go on to elaborate and give related examples in the rest of the paragraph.
- Try to link your paragraphs so that the text reads logically. If you put ten different ideas in ten different paragraphs and do not connect them in any way, the reader may think you are talking about many disconnected ideas.
- You could try to link the paragraph above to the one below by writing something related to the next paragraph in the last sentence of the paragraph before.
- While writing keep your reader's needs in mind. This means providing a verbal 'map' of your document so that your reader knows what to expect, and placing verbal 'signposts' in your text to explain what is coming next.

Key points

- Plan and structure the discussion section of your review.
- Start your discussion with a summary of your findings in words.
- Ensure that you discuss all the results you presented in the results section:
  - discuss the results of the studies you selected based on the title and abstract and based on reading the full paper
  - discuss your included studies in terms of PICO or PEO
  - discuss the quality of your included studies in a synthesized format
  - provide a detailed discussion of the data extracted.
- Develop and/or discuss any theory or theories as to how the intervention (or exposure) works.
- Compare and contrast the findings of your study.
- Relate the findings back to the objectives set out and the initial area of interest.
- Make recommendations on how these shortcomings may be rectified in future.
- Discuss the findings with respect to practice and/or policy.
- Discuss the ethical aspects of the included studies.
- Reveal questions for future research on this topic.
- Finish your discussion by stating some overall conclusions about the study.
- Provide overall conclusions about your review.
- Write up your systematic review to a high standard (this is a fundamental part of the systematic literature review process).
- Take as much care in writing up the review as in conducting the review.

- Ensure that you include all aspects of the systematic review process in the:
  - background
  - objectives
  - inclusion and exclusion criteria
  - methods of selecting your papers
  - appraisal of your papers
  - extraction of relevant data
  - results section
  - discussion section
  - conclusions.
- Finally, take great care over the presentation of your review: check your spelling, grammar and syntax.

Summary

This chapter discussed ways of structuring the discussion section of your systematic literature review. Extracts from case studies and a completed systematic review were presented. Suggestions for writing up your review report were described together with tips for improving academic writing skills.

Question and Answer (Q&A)

(Q) What are the benefits of systematic reviews?

(A) There are several benefits in undertaking systematic reviews. They have the potential to inform policy-makers, commissioners, professionals and the public with reliable sources of evidence. They support academics and researchers in identifying gaps in the knowledge surrounding a particular area and or specialty. They are effective in summarizing findings from the vast amounts of literature. They can help to improve patient care and the working environments for staff.

12

Checking your systematic review is complete and some practical ways to share and disseminate your findings

Overview

- PRISMA statement
- Systematic review checklist
- Practical ways to help support you in sharing and disseminating your systematic review

We have decided to include this chapter as most of our students conducting a systematic review found it very useful to be able to check that they had included all necessary steps essential to conducting a good systematic review once they had finished their dissertation. When we were teaching our undergraduate BSc and postgraduate MSc students how to conduct a systematic review for their dissertation some lecturers also used this checklist to mark their students' dissertations. This checklist could also be used to check other authors' systematic reviews to assess whether or not the reviews have included all the relevant sections and addressed them appropriately. We have also included a section offering some practical ways to help support you in sharing and disseminating your systematic review.

PRISMA statement

Before we go any further we would just like to say a word about the PRISMA (preferred reporting items for systematic reviews and meta-analysis) statement that many of you may have heard about already. This statement was developed by a group of 29 review authors, methodologists, clinicians, medical editors and consumers. A Delphi consensus process was used to develop a 27-item checklist (http://www.prisma-statement. org/) and a four-phase flow diagram (see Figure12.1). The aim of the consensus was to agree on the items that most authors deemed were essential for the transparent reporting of a systematic review. After 11 revisions these authors approved the checklist, flow diagram and an explanatory paper that has been published numerous times in different journals and websites to make sure it was disseminated as widely as possible (Moher et al. 2009). You may find that a number of items on our checklist are similar to the ones included within the PRISMA statement. However, our checklist was developed many years before the PRISMA statement and was developed primarily with the aim of helping students make sure their systematic review is complete.

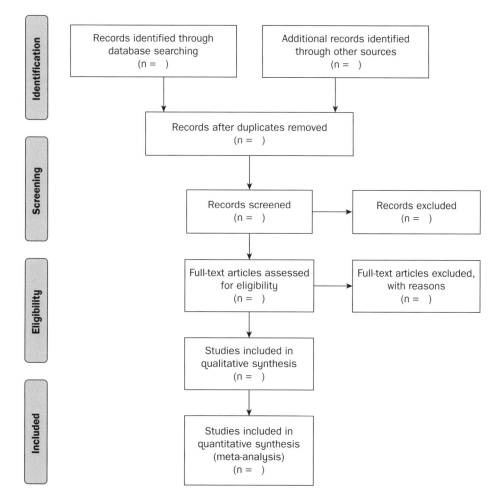

Figure 12.1 PRISMA 2009 flow diagram.

From: Moher D, Liberati A, Tetzlaff J, Altman DG,The PRISMA Group (2009). Preferred Reporting Items for Systematic Reviews and Meta-Analyses: The PRISMA Statement. *PLoS Med 6 (6)*: e1000097. doi:10.1371/journal.pmed100009.

Systematic review checklist

The systematic review checklist provided in Table 12.1 offers a comprehensive overview of what should be included in your systematic review.

Practical Tip

If your read and review the systematic review checklist prior to commencing your review you will be more confident and aware of what you need to do to conduct a systematic literature review and how to go about undertaking your own review.

Table 12. 1 Systematic review (SR) checklist

Title and question of the SR	Commentary/explanation	Example of possible responses
1 Is the title a true representation of the content?	Essentially what you are checking for is to see if the content of the SR is truly what the title says. For instance having completed your SR, does the title include the words 'systematic review' within it? A good way to include this is to write your title as a statement and then put a colon and add 'systematic review' after this, for example 'Comparison of surgical versus non-surgical interventions for adolescent patients with scoliosis: A systematic review'. Note: if you are writing a SR for Cochrane, however, it is slightly different as they have their own format for writing the titles.	√
2 Has an appropriate question relevant to the area of expertise been developed?	Have you developed an appropriate research question and title for your SR? And is it within your or the authors' area of expertise?	√
3 Are all components of the question (PICO or PEO) included within the title?	Are all the PICO or PEO components written within the title and are these clear and easy to find?	? ?
If the SR is not your own please check questions 4 and 5. If it is your own SR that you are checking please make sure that you are credible and have no conflicts of interest.		
4 Are the authors credible? Do they appear to have the appropriate qualifications to write a SR in this area?	Do the authors appear to be appropriately qualified in this field from what you can read in the SR? The best way to check for this is to see what professions and qualifications the authors have by looking at the letters after their names as well as their place of work.	X

5   Is it clear from what you have read that the authors have no conflict of interest?

This is very important to check as if the authors have a conflict of interest then there is a possibility that the results of the SR may be biased. So for instance if the authors were part of a company that made braces then their SR may be biased towards the effectiveness of this intervention.

Comments:

Abstract of the SR

6   Is there a clear summary of the research? This should include the background, objectives (and rationale), inclusion and exclusion criteria, search strategy, methods, results, conclusions and implications for the field. Abstract ideally to be no more than 350–500 words.

Here you just need to check whether all the sections are included and make sure to count the number of words in your abstract. This may vary depending on the actual criteria for your dissertation, or if you are submitting it to a journal the word count may differ depending on the instructions to authors for that particular journal.

7   Is the abstract structured? If so are all the sections included within the full SR included and described?

The abstract or summary of your SR needs to contain a description of each section of the full review. What we usually recommend to students conducting this type of dissertation is to write a structured abstract. What this means is that the abstract should contain the same subheadings as those contained within the full SR. In other words the following subheadings: the background, objectives (and rationale), inclusion and exclusion criteria, search strategy, methods, results, discussion and conclusions. In this way it will make it easy for you not to leave anything out. What we have found over and over again is that if the abstract is not structured that students will tend to leave one or more sections out.

Table 12. 1 Continued

8	If unstructured - are all sections of the SR included and described?	If you need to go with an unstructured abstract then do make sure all the sections have been included. We have found from teaching hundreds of students to conduct SR dissertations that a common pitfall is to write an overview (in other words a more general abstract that does not give the specific details of each section that are actually needed).

Chapter 1: Background

9	Is the Introduction to the area well written and would it be considered capable of promoting interest?	Within the introduction it is important to highlight the importance of the topic within the context within which it is used. As discussed in the protocol chapter you need to check that you have included statistics as well as key government documents to highlight how this topic or clinical condition is currently of great importance for patients and other readers.
10	Is there an explanation of how the review extends the existing literature? Or if it is a duplication of another review is it clear how the student's review is different?	For this section you are essentially checking how the review is extending what is already known. In other words is this SR original? And if so what other SRs have been conducted in a similar field and how is your review extending the current knowledge? Is it clear how your review differs to what is already out there?
11	Relevance of the study to the field or gap in knowledge i.e. the student needs to show that no review exactly like theirs has been carried out.	When you highlight the SRs that have already been conducted within this area it is crucial to highlight what these reviews have and have not addressed. The key point here is to very clearly show what is currently missing within these reviews and this should take you very nicely to clarifying the gap in the literature that your own review will address.

| 12 | Does it demonstrate some knowledge of the specialist area of practice? And does it question orthodox practice using balanced, logical and supported argument? (This part needs to be continued in much more depth in the discussion.) | Part of item 12 is generally addressed within the background section and then the rest of this discussion is addressed within the discussion section. |
| 13 | Is independence of thought and open-mindedness demonstrated? | It is very important to make sure that you are expressing your own opinions and critical skills and not just taking all you read in other papers at face value. |

Comments:

Chapter 2: Objectives

14	Statement of the study's objective/s (or if relevant hypotheses).	As mentioned previously in this book it is important that the objectives are very similar or identical to the title. Do make sure that your objectives also include all the PICO or PEO elements, as does the title.
15	Are the objectives (or research question) based on the background?	Do make sure that your title and the background are very closely linked.
16	Is it clear how these objectives will be measured?	Make sure that this is stated clearly especially in the inclusion and exclusion criteria section.
17	Are they relevant to the clinical area under investigation?	Just a yes or no answer is required here with the rationale.
18	Are they clear, conscience and comprehensive reflecting the title	Just a yes or no answer is required with the rationale.

Chapter 3: Criteria for considering studies in review

| 19 | Have details of the types of participants to be included in the review been described? | In this section it is important to include who your population is, their clinical diagnosis, their gender, age range, time since diagnosis, together with your rationale – as well as who you will be excluding and why. |
| 20 | Have details been given of the types of intervention to be included in review? | Make sure that within this section you have clearly stated and described the intervention/s that you were including in your SR. |

Table 12. 1 Continued

21	Have details been given of the types of comparative groups to be included in the review?	Same as above but for the comparative intervention. Tip: do make it very clear what the similarities and differences are between the intervention and comparative interventions.
22	Have details been given of the types of outcome measures to be included in the review?	It is important for you to very clearly specify precisely what outcome measures were included and how these were to be measured. This should include units of measurement, i.e. whether the outcomes in question are measured for instance in degrees or centimetres, etc.
23	Have details been given of the types of study (designs) to be included in the review?	Once again this is very important to specify. In this section you should have mentioned whether your SR only included randomized controlled trials (RCTs) or controlled clinical trials (CCTs) or cohort studies or just case studies (if for instance research in a particular field is very limited) or all quantitative or all qualitative studies etc. In the event that you are conducting a mixed SR then it would be appropriate to include both qualitative and quantitative designs.

Chapter 4: Search strategy

24	Were all databases searched described?	When writing down the databases that you have searched do make sure that you have described the name of the database together with the dates in years that it covers.

25	Was the search strategy based on components of the review question?	It is very important that within the search strategy section of your SR you describe how you developed the search strategy from the actual research question and that your search strategy includes *all components* of the SR question.
26	Were all possible sources of literature searched? e.g. electronic databases, MEDLINE, EMBASE, PsychLIT, CINAHL, etc?	In order for your search strategy to be as clear, comprehensive and transparent as possible all the databases together with the years they covered need to be listed. This includes the two sections below as well, checking specialist trial registers and hand searching.
27	Were specialist trial registers checked: Cochrane?	Yes, No, Unclear
28	Was hand searching undertaken?	Yes, No, Unclear
29	Were reference lists checked?	All references of all the papers you decided to include within the SR need to have been checked. Usually many similar papers can be found in this way.
30	Was any grey literature checked? for example, PhDs and BScs in libraries, conference proceedings or abstracts?	Do make sure you have remembered to include the grey literature. This includes for example PhD theses and conference abstracts that have not as yet been published but that are still necessary for you to include within your SR.
31	Was the description of the search strategy detailed enough to the extent that someone else could duplicate it and get the same results?	In the same way that a primary study needs to be able to be replicated, the search strategy needs to be listed and reported in such a way that a colleague of average intelligence could replicate it.

Table 12. 1 Continued

32	Were the numbers of papers located at each step of the search mentioned?	In order to make sure you have followed this advice many students and researchers use a flow chart to document each step of the search. If you look at most Cochrane reviews, they all include one. Please refer to page XX and Figure 12.1 to see what this looks like.
33	Overall was the search efficient and used appropriately?	Here you need to check that the search terms and synonyms are actually derived from the research question and that the terms have been combined appropriately using Boolean terms of AND and OR.
34	Have details of all three parts of the methods section been described?	For this item you just need to check that all three parts of the methods section (i.e. selecting, evaluating the quality of your papers or evaluating the risk of bias, data extracting) have been included.

Chapter 5 Methods

Stage 1: Study selection
The process of selecting papers for inclusion in the review (this process consists of two steps: the initial paper selection followed by the second more thorough selection of papers)

 Step 1 of study selection

| 35 | Was the first selection of papers (for inclusion in review) based on titles and abstracts only? | This item is self-explanatory. When checking that you have both conducted and reported this do make sure that it is clearly reported within your dissertation or paper. Ideally you should have included a subheading stating 'first selection of papers based on titles and abstracts'. |

36	Did the student conduct it alone or did two students perform it independently? If alone did they state that this might affect (or have an impact) on both the reliability and the validity of the papers selected? (you may hear this referred to as selection bias in other papers or books).	You will find that SRs conducted within Cochrane, the Campbell Collaboration or the Joanna Briggs Institute are conducted by more than one author who will conduct the methods section (selection of papers, evaluation of methodological quality or bias) independently and then compare the results between them. This is done to increase the validity of these processes. If you are doing this SR for a dissertation, however, you will probably be conducting it on your own. This is fine too but it is important that you have mentioned within your own SR that because you have done the SR on your own the methods section may not be as reliable and valid.
37	Were the procedures to be used tested on a sample of articles (somewhat like a pilot study)?	Like in a primary study it is important to conduct a pilot study on a few of the papers using the standardized forms just to make sure that they work well and that you have included everything you need to select your papers and extract data from them.
38	Was a standardized form made for this procedure? Is it appropriate and adequate to answer the research question?	Here you need to check that the standardized form you created actually answers fully your research question.
39	Was a clear description provided of the criteria the students were looking for at this stage?	For this item you need to check that all the inclusion and exclusion criteria for all aspects of PICOT or PEOT have been included within your SR.

Table 12. 1 Continued

40	Was it clear how disagreements were resolved?	For this item you need to check that you have stated how the two independent reviewers were selected and how they conducted the selection and review of the paper. If the two independent reviewers could not reach agreement on the review then it should be made clear how an additional author was selected to conduct the review process.
41	Did the student state how many papers were included initially and how many papers were left after the initial first selection?	Again please make sure that you have stated how many papers were included initially and how many papers were left after the initial first selection.
42	Were reasons provided for the papers that were discarded?	This item is self-explanatory.
43	Is it clear how disagreements were resolved?	This item is self-explanatory.

 Step 2 of study selection (more thorough selection of papers)

44	The criteria for this section are the same as above except that the selection of papers is based on reading the whole paper.	This item is self-explanatory.

Stage 2: The procedure for the assessment of methodological quality

45	Was the appropriate checklist used to assess the methodological quality of each paper included in the study? e.g. if student used RCTs, CCTs and qualitative papers, then three checklists need to be included and described in this section.	As you may already know there are numerous checklists for various types of research designs. For this item it is important to check that if you had a variety of research designs, that you have used the right checklist for that type of design. The Caldwell checklist is easy as you can use the same checklist to assess the quality of all your research papers.

46	Were the checklists or evaluation documents used appropriately and were they well cited and referenced?	Usually the documents for this item are placed in the appendix where your supervisor can check that you have filled in your checklists appropriately. It will ultimately help you to take some more time and use a book or explanatory guide to help you fill in the checklist items appropriately.
47	Was it clear how many people assessed the studies and how this was carried out?	The purpose of this item is to *assess* how valid your results are. Obviously if two independent assessments have been made by two students of the same papers the results will be more valid and less prone to error than if you conducted this process on your own. But as we said previously if you did conduct it on your own you need to mention it as a limitation of your study.
48	Were assessments done independently? If not did you state the effect this might have on the results of the evaluation of the studies.	As above.
49	Was a description given of how the papers were evaluated? (e.g. poor, adequate, good, very good, excellent? Or was a more objective numerical method used?)	The Cochrane Collaboration does not actually use a numerical scale. They call the methodological evaluation the 'risk of bias' with greater risk being found in poor studies or studies lower down on the hierarchy of evidence. So RCTs will have a low risk of bias and a case study will have a high risk of bias.

Stage3: The data extraction strategy

50	Was the appropriate data extracted to enable the research question to be answered?	When checking this item it is important to make sure that you have extracted data for each part of the review question i.e. PICOT and that these are clear for a reader to understand and interpret.

Table 12. 1 Continued

51	Was the standardized form used to extract data, appropriate to collect all the data necessary to answer the research question?	It is important to make sure you include all the data extraction forms in the appendix of your dissertation. If you are conducting the SR for publication in a paper then it is not necessary to show this work, however, we would suggest you keep them in case you need them while the paper is being reviewed.
52	Was the data extraction form piloted in any way before it was used in the study?	Again do make sure this is clearly mentioned in the appropriate section of your SR.
53	Was data extracted by more than one student/reviewer?	As explained above.
54	How were disagreements resolved?	As explained above.

Chapter 6: Data synthesis (results)

Were all 6 sections of the results included (very important)?

55	Were the results of the search included and presented?	This item is self-explanatory. Ideally the results of your search can either be presented in a table or better still in the freely available template (Figure 1) available from the PRISMA website.
56	Were all the results of the studies selected based on the title and abstract clearly presented?	This item is self-explanatory. Please see the chapter on Synthesizing, summarizing and presenting your results for a full explanation of this.
57	Were the results of the included studies based on reading the full paper presented?	Please see the chapter on Synthesizing, summarizing and presenting your results for a full explanation of this.
58	Was a summary of all the included studies within your SR presented and were all PICOT parts included?	Please see the chapter on Synthesizing, summarizing and presenting your results for a full explanation of this.
59	Was a summary of all the critiques of the papers using the appropriate frameworks included?	This item is self-explanatory. Please see the chapter on Synthesizing, summarizing and presenting your results for a full explanation of this.

60	Was a summary of the data extracted presented? (including a synthesis of the overall results)?	Please see the chapter on Synthesizing, summarizing and presenting your results for a full explanation of this.
61	Were the results presented in an effective format?	Please see the chapter on Synthesizing, summarizing and presenting your results for a full explanation of this.
62	Was the presentation of tables and/or figures clear and complete?	Please see the chapter on Synthesizing, summarizing and presenting your results for a full explanation of this.
63	Was duplication of data presentation avoided?	This item is self-explanatory. Please see the chapter on Synthesizing, summarizing and presenting your results for a full explanation of this.
64	Was text used to clarify trends within the data?	This item is self-explanatory. Please see the chapter on Synthesizing, summarizing and presenting your results for a full explanation of this.
65	Was the data appropriately synthesized?	This item is self-explanatory. Please see the chapter on Synthesizing, summarizing and presenting your results for a full explanation of this.
66	Were the standardized forms on which all the data was collected included in the appendix? Were they appropriately filled in? (this item is for dissertations only)	This item is self-explanatory.

Chapter 7: Discussion and conclusions

67	Does the student demonstrate a comprehensive and detailed knowledge of the specialist area of practice and question orthodox practice using balanced, logical and supported argument (continued from background)?	This item is self-explanatory.
68	Was the interpretation of the results discussed with respect to theory, research literature, practice and ethics?	This item is self-explanatory.

Table 12. 1 Continued

69	Was the overall quality of the included studies discussed?	This item is self-explanatory.
70	Were the implications of the review discussed?	This item is self-explanatory.
71	Were the major deficiencies of the review discussed?	This item is self-explanatory.
72	Were the conclusions and the main relevant findings clearly summarized?	This item is self-explanatory.
73	Were recommendations made for future research and/or reviews?	This item is self-explanatory.

References

74	Was the Harvard format used?	This item is self-explanatory.
75	Do citations and references match?	This item is self-explanatory.
76	Are the references accurately presented?	This item is self-explanatory.
77	Did you include a wide range and scope of papers?	This item is self-explanatory.

Presentation

78	Was the correct layout used for title page, contents, page numbers, etc. (see these guidelines)?	This item is self-explanatory.
79	Is the text free from errors and spelling mistakes?	This item is self-explanatory.
80	Is there appropriate use of vocabulary and grammar?	This item is self-explanatory.
81	Is there appropriate use of the appendices?	This item is self-explanatory.
82	Is there a logical and clear presentation of appendices?	This item is self-explanatory.
83	Is there a clear and aesthetic style and presentation of the report as a whole?	This item is self-explanatory.

Overall comments:

Key to possible responses on the systematic review checklist

√ This sign shows you have included the item and addressed it appropriately.

? This sign suggests that you are not sure whether you have or have not addressed the item correctly and/or in sufficient detail. You will need to go back to your paper/dissertation to check whether or not you have included it and sufficiently addressed this issue.

X This sign shows that you have not included this item or you have not addressed it correctly. You will need to go back to this item in your thesis or paper and amend your work.

We hope that by providing this systematic review checklist you will be able to cross-reference your own systematic review to make sure that you have included all the required aspects for submitting a good review. Once all the aspects are complete students can consider whether to share or publish their systematic review. From our experiences we find that many of our undergraduate and postgraduate students are satisfied with submitting their completed review only for their relevant degree. They prefer to leave things here, which is fine. The thought of doing any more work and/or publishing their work seems to be a bridge too far. For some of our students confidence is often the issue and the thought of having your work firstly marked and then possibly peer-reviewed is a daunting prospect, which we do acknowledge and appreciate.

We do, however, actively encourage our students to think about sharing and disseminating their work in order to improve practice. The next section offers some practical ways to help support you in sharing and disseminating your review should you decide to do this once the review is complete.

Practical ways to help support you in sharing and disseminating your systematic review

There are numerous articles and books offering sound information and advice about the opportunities and challenges associated with sharing and disseminating research findings and how this is important to ensure that we practise using an evidence base. The failure to share and disseminate the findings from research and or systematic reviews could have an impact on the following:

- building a knowledge and evidence base for nursing and midwifery
- informing healthcare managers, leaders and policy-makers
- establishing impact and outcomes of care
- offering equity through knowledge exchange and translation
- advancing innovation and change.

Lavis et al. (2005: 35) suggest 'that systematic reviews of research evidence constitute a more appropriate source of research evidence for decision-making than the latest or most heavily publicized research study'. This is because the dissemination of the results and findings from original research and systematic reviews can contribute to the following:

- adding new knowledge to the field
- evaluating specific nursing interventions and practices
- focusing on improving the quality of nursing and midwifery care and interventions and associated patient outcomes
- helping services to adopt and implement innovation
- supporting the practising of evidence-based nursing.

Despite all the evidence highlighting the importance of sharing and disseminating the findings from original research and systematic reviews to improve the quality of nursing care, interventions and outcomes, why do some researchers not publish their findings? Timmins (2015) offers some useful and practical guidance on why some nursing research does not find its way to improve practice and inform decision-making. A key statement from Timmins (2015: 43) is the following: 'research undertaken by nurses, or in the domain of nursing, is not likely to be used by others unless it is useful to nurses and support is provided for it to be implemented in practice'. Two important words from Timmins' statement stand out for us when focusing on the importance of sharing and disseminating findings from research: 'useful' and 'support'.

We believe that when focusing on sharing and disseminating the findings from research and or systematic reviews that the researcher thinks about the following. 'Sharing' is defined as 'to receive, use, in common with others' and 'dissemination' is 'to scatter far and wide' (Collins 1987). If you focus on sharing your work by making it 'useful', accessible and easy to read, and seek 'support' from supervisors, colleagues and journal editors to ensure your research findings are shared widely, we could see fruit in terms of further improvements in care and services. This is because nurses and midwives will be more comfortable about reading, reviewing and taking action on the findings and recommendations from your work.

The Centre for Reviews and Dissemination (2008) defines dissemination as the:

> Planned and active process that seeks to ensure that those who need to know about a piece of research get to know about it and can make sense of the findings. As such it involves more than making research accessible through traditional mediums of academic journals and conference presentation.
>
> (Centre for Reviews and Dissemination 2008: 85)

We would suggest that an effective strategy and action plan for sharing and disseminating your findings from a systematic review should focus on achieving the following.

- Ensuring that the essential message(s) from the findings reach the specific target audience(s) associated with the area of practice reviewed.
- Providing the findings in a format or style that is both accessible and relevant to frontline nurses and midwives.

Having identified a strategy and action plan for the sharing and dissemination of your findings it is important to identify some possible ways to publish your findings. Taylor (2014) *Chapter 10 - Disseminating your work: presentations and conferences* and *Chapter 11 – Disseminating knowledge through publication* offers some great practical advice and guidance to support you in disseminating your work.

Practical Tip

If everyone who undertakes nursing research and a systematic review decide not to publish their work how will the nursing profession continue to improve for the future? By publishing your work you are contributing to furthering the profession.

We would suggest that to achieve evidence-based nursing, you need to be evidence-informed, which involves:

Providing clinically effective patient care and being able to justify the procedures used, the care plan devised or the services provided by reference to authoritative evidence. It is the making of decisions about the care of individual patients and families, on the basis of the best available evidence.

(McSherry et al. 2002: 3)

To ensure that we are all evidence-informed the challenge for those who have undertaken a systematic review is in devising a strategy for the sharing and dissemination of your research findings. This is important in order to inform the evidence base of nursing.

Key points

- Check that you have included all necessary steps essential to conducting a good systematic review once you have finished your review and/or dissertation.
- The systematic review checklist offers a compressive overview of what should be included in your systematic review.
- By providing the systematic review checklist you will be able to cross-reference that you have included all the required aspects for your review.
- We would actively encourage you to think about sharing and disseminating your work in order to improve practice.
- Devising an effective strategy and action plan for the sharing and dissemination of your findings from your systematic review will aid publication.

Summary

The chapter provides a detailed systematic review checklist and some practical advice and guidance on how and why it is important to consider sharing and disseminating the findings from your review.

Question and Answer (Q&A)

(Q) Who are the users of systematic reviews?

(A) The findings from systematic reviews can be used by a variety and diversity of stakeholders. These include doctors, nurses, researchers, policy-makers, patients, commissioners and insurers, to name but a few.

References

Abdullah, G., Rossy, D., Ploeg, J., et al. (2014) Measuring the effectiveness of mentoring as a knowledge translation intervention for implementing empirical evidence: a systematic review. *Worldviews on Evidence-Based Nursing* 11 (5): 284–300.

Armstrong, R., Jackson, N., Doyle, J., Waters, E. and Howes, F. (2005) It's in your hands: The value of handsearching in conducting systematic reviews of public health interventions. *Journal of Public Health* 27 (4): 388–391. Available at http://jpubhealth.oxfordjournals.org/cgi/content/abstract/27/4/388 (accessed 6 November 2015).

Asher, M., Min, L.S., Burton, D. and Manna, B. (2003) The reliability and concurrent validity of the Scoliosis Research Society-22 patient questionnaire for idiopathic scoliosis. *Spine* 28 (1): 63–69.

Bailey, D.M. (1997) *Research for the Health Professional: A Practical Guide*, 2nd edn. Philadelphia, PA: F.A. Davis.

Blaikie, N. (2007) *Approaches to Social Enquiry*, 2nd edn. Cambridge: Polity Press.

Bruce, N., Pope, D. and Stanistreet, D. (2008) *Quantitative Methods for Health Research: A Practical Interactive Guide to Epidemiology and Statistics*. London: Wiley.

Burnard, P. (1991) A method of analysing interview transcripts in qualitative research. *Nurse Education Today* 11 (6): 461–466.

Caldwell, K., Henshaw, L. and Taylor, G. (2011) Developing a framework for critiquing health research: An early evaluation. *Nurse Education Today* 31 (8): e1–7.

Centre for Evidence-Based Medicine (2015) *EBM Resources*. Oxford: CEBM. Available at http://www.cebm.net/ (accessed 13 November 2015).

Centre for Reviews and Dissemination (CRD) (2008) *Systematic Reviews: CRD's Guidance for Undertaking Reviews in Health Care*. Available at http://www.york.ac.uk/crd/guidance/ (accessed 24 September 2015).

Cochrane Collaboration (2009) *Cochrane Handbook for Systematic Reviews of Interventions*. Available at www.cochrane-handbook.org (accessed 24 September 2015).

Cochrane Collaboration (2014) *Cochrane Reviews*. London: Cochrane Collaboration. Available at http://community.cochrane.org/cochrane-reviews (accessed 13 November 2015).

Cochrane Effective Practice and Organization of Care (2011) *Cochrane Effective Practice and Organization of Care (EPOC) Group*. Available at http://epoc.cochrane.org (accessed 24 September 2015).

Collins, W. (1987) *Collins Universal English Dictionary*. Glasgow: Readers Union.

Craig, J. and Smyth, R.L. (2002) *The Evidence-Based Practice Manual for Nurses*. London: Churchill Livingstone.

Craig, J. and Smyth, R.L. (2007) *The Evidence-Based Practice Manual for Nurses*, 2nd edn. London: Churchill Livingstone.

de Brito, M. and Gommes, B. (2015) Non-cancer palliative care in the community needs greater interprofessional collaboration to maintain coordinated care and manage uncertainty. *Evidence-Based Nursing* 18 (3): 79.

DiCenso, A., Cullum, N. and Ciliska, D. (1998) Implementing evidence-based nursing: Some misconceptions. *Evidence-Based Nursing* 1 (2): 38–40.

Dickersin, K., Chan, S., Chalmers, T.C., Sacks, H.S. and Smith, H. (1987) Publication bias and clinical trials. *Controlled Clinical Trials* 8 (4): 343–353.

Docherty, M. and Smith, R. (1999) The case for structuring the discussion of scientific papers. *British Medical Journal* 318: 1224.

Douglas, R.M., Hemilä, H., Chalker, E. and Treacy, B. (2004) Vitamin C for preventing and treating the common cold. *Cochrane Database of Systematic Reviews* CD000980.

Egger, M., Zellweger-Zähner, T., Schneider, M., Junker, C., Lengeler, G. and Antes, G. (1997) Language bias in randomized controlled trials published in English and German. *The Lancet* 350 (9074): 326–329.

Field, P.A. and Morse, J.M. (1985) *Nursing Research: The Application of Qualitative Approaches*. London: Chapman and Hall.

Flemming, K. (1998) Asking answerable questions. *Evidence-Based Nursing* 1: 36–37.

Glaser, B.G. and Strauss, A. (1967) *Discovery of Grounded Theory. Strategies for Qualitative Research*. Mill Valley, CA: Sociology Press.

Glasziou, P., Irwig, L., Bain, C. and Colditz, G. (2001) *Systematic Reviews in Health Care: A Practical Guide*. Cambridge: Cambridge University Press.

Goodenough, T.J. and Brysiewicz, P. (2003) Witnessed resuscitation – Exploring the attitudes and practices of the emergency staff working in Level 1 Emergency Departments in the province of KwaZulu-Natal. *Curationis* 26 (2): 56–63.

Greene, M. (1997) The lived world, literature and education. In D. Vandenberg (ed.) *Phenomenology and Educational Discourse*. Johannesburg: Heinemann.

Health and Care Professions Council (2012) *Standards of Conduct, Performance and Ethics*. London: Health and Care Professions Council. Available at http://www.hpc-uk.org/aboutreg istration/standards/standardsofconductperformanceandethics/ (accessed 13 November 2015).

Hemmingway, P. and Brereton, N. (2009) *What is a Systematic Review?* Available at http:// www.medicine.ox.ac.uk/bandolier/painres/download/whatis/syst-review.pdf (accessed 6 November 2015).

Higgins, J.P.T. and Deeks, J. (2009) *Cochrane Handbook for Systematic Reviews of Interventions*. London: The Cochrane Collaboration. Available at http://handbook.cochrane.org/v5.0.2/ (accessed 5 November 2015).

Higgins, J.P.T. and Green, S. (2011). *Cochrane Handbook for Systematic Reviews of Interventions Version 5.1.0* (updated March 2011). London: The Cochrane Collaboration. Available at www.cochrane-handbook.org (accessed 23 November 2015).

Jadad, A. (1998) *Randomized Controlled Trials: A User's Guide*. London: BMJ Books.

Jenkins, S., Price, C.J. and Straker, L. (1998) *The Researching Therapist: A Practical Guide to Planning, Performing and Communicating Research*. Edinburgh: Churchill Livingstone.

Khan, K.S., Kunz, R., Kleijnen, J. and Antes, G. (2003) *Systematic Reviews to Support Evidence-Based Medicine: How to Review and Apply Findings of Healthcare Research*. London: Royal Society of Medicine Press.

Knott, A. and Kee, C.C. (2005) Nurses' beliefs about family presence during resuscitation. *Applied Nursing Research* 18: 192–198.

Lahlafi, A. (2007) Conducting a literature review: How to carry out bibliographical database searches. *British Journal of Cardiac Nursing* 2 (12): 566–569.

Lai, S.M., Asher, M. and Burton, D. (2006) Estimating SRS-22 quality of life measures with SF-36: Application in idiopathic scoliosis. *Spine* 31 (4): 473–478.

Lavis, J., Davies, H., Oxman, A., Denis, J.L., Goldend-Biddle, K. and Ferlie, E. (2005) Towards systematic reviews that inform healthcare management and policy making. *Journal of Health Service Research and Policy* 1 (1): 35–48.

Law, M., Steward, D., Pollock, N., Letts, L., Bosch, J. and Westmorland, M. (1998) *Critical Review Form – Quantitative Studies*. Ontario: The McMaster University. Available at http://www.srs-mcmaster.ca/ (accessed 12 November 2015).

McCormack, H.M., Horne, D.J. and Sheather, S. (1988) Clinical applications of visual analogue scales: A critical review. *Psychological Medicine* 18 (4): 1007–1019.

McSherry, R., Simmons, M. and Abbott, P. (eds) (2002) *Evidence-Informed Nursing: A Guide for Clinical Nurses*. London: Routledge.

Moher, D., Liberati, A., Tetzlaff, J., Altman, D.G. and the PRISMA Group (2009) Preferred Reporting Items for Systematic reviews and Meta-Analyses: The PRISMA Statement. *British Medical Journal* 339: bmj.b2535. Available at www.bmj.com/content/339/bmj.b2535.full?view=long&pmid=19622551 (accessed 6 November 2015).

National Institute for Health Research (NIHR) (2010) *Systematic Reviews: Knowledge to Support Evidence Informed Health and Social Care*. London: NIHR. Available at http://docplayer.net/6808443-Systematic-reviews-knowledge-to-support-evidence-informed-health-and-so cial-care.html (accessed 13 November 2015).

Negrini, S., Minozzi, S., Bettany-Saltikov, J., et al. (2010) Braces for idiopathic scoliosis in adolescents. *Cochrane Database of Systematic Reviews* CD006850. Available at http://onlinelibrary.wiley.com/doi/10.1002/14651858.CD006850.pub2/pdf (accessed 6 November 2015).

Negrini, S., Minozzi, S., Bettany-Saltikov, J., et al. (2015) Braces for idiopathic scoliosis in adolescents. *Cochrane Database of Systematic Reviews* CD006850. Available at http://onlinelibrary.wiley.com/doi/10.1002/14651858.CD006850.pub3/abstract (accessed 23 November 2015).

NHS Institute for Innovation and Improvement (2010) *High Impact Actions for Nursing and Midwifery: The Essential Collection*. Coventry: NHS Institute for Innovation and Improvement. Available at http://www.institute.nhs.uk/building_capability/general/aims/ (accessed 13 November 2015).

Noyes, J., Popay, J., Pearson, A., Hannes, K. and Booth, A. (2008) Qualitative research and Cochrane reviews. In J.P.T. Higgins and S. Green (eds) *Cochrane Handbook for Systematic Reviews of Interventions. Version 5.0.1* (updated September 2008). Cochrane Collaboration. Available at www.cochrane-handbook.org (accessed 24 September 2015).

Nursing and Midwifery Council (2004) *The NMC Code of Professional Conduct: Standards for Conduct, Performance and Ethics*. London: NMC.

Nursing and Midwifery Council (2015) *The Code: Professional Standards of Practice and Behaviour for Nurses and Midwives*. London: Nursing and Midwifery Council. Available at http://www.nmc.org.uk/standards/code/ (accessed 13 November 2015).

O'Brien, J.A. and Fothergill-Bourbonnais, F. (2004) The experience of trauma resuscitation in the emergency department: Themes from seven patients. *Journal of Emergency Nursing* 30 (3): 216–224.

Pauling, L. (1974) Are recommended daily allowances for vitamin C adequate? *Proceedings of the National Academy of Sciences of the United States of America* 71 (11): 4442–4446.

Petticrew, M. and Roberts, H. (2006) *Systematic Reviews in the Social Sciences: A Practical Guide*. Oxford: Blackwell.

Polit, D.F. and Beck, C.T. (2006) *Essentials of Nursing Research: Methods, Appraisal, and Utilization*. Philadelphia: Lippincott Williams & Wilkins.

Popay, J., Roberts, H., Sowden, A., et al. (2006) *Guidance on the Conduct of Narrative Synthesis in Systematic Reviews*, Version 1. Lancaster: Lancaster University.

Roe, B. (2015) Systematic review of systematic reviews for the management of urinary incontinence and promotion of continence using conservative behavioural approaches in older people in care homes. *Journal of Advanced Nursing* 71 (7): 1464–1483.

Rooda, L.A. (1994) Effects of mind mapping on student achievement in a nursing research course. *Nurse Educator* 19 (6): 25–27.

Sackett, D.L., Richardson, W.S., Rosenberg, W. and Haynes, R.B. (1997) *Evidence-Based Medicine: How to Practice and Teach EBM*. New York: Churchill Livingston.

Schulz, K.F. and Grimes, D.A. (2002) Case-control studies: Research in reverse. *The Lancet* 359 (9304): 431–434.

Scoliosis Research Society (SRS) (2006). *Common Questions and Glossary*. Scoliosis Research Society. Available at www.srs.org/ (accessed 24 September 2015).

Spradley, J.P. (1979) *The Ethnographic Interview*. New York: Holt, Rinehart and Winston.

Taylor, B.D. (2014) *Writing Skills in Nursing and Healthcare: A Guide to Completing Successful Dissertations and Theses*. London: Sage Publications.

Timmermans, S. (1997) High touch in high tech: The presence of relatives and friends during resuscitative efforts. *Scholarly Inquiry for Nursing Practice* 11 (2): 154–168.

Timmins, F. (2015) Disseminating nursing research. *Nursing Standard* 29 (48): 34–39.

Timmins, F. and McCabe, C. (2005) How to conduct an effective literature search. *Nursing Standard* 20 (11): 41–47.

Tingle, J. and Cribb, A. (eds) (2002) *Nursing Law and Ethics*, 2nd edn. Oxford: Blackwell.

Torgerson, C. (2003) *Systematic Reviews*. London: Continuum.

Weiss, H.R., Reichel, D., Schanz, J. and Zimmermann-Gudd, S. (2006) Deformity related stress in adolescents with AIS. *Studies in Health Technology and Informatics* 123: 347–351.

Index